I'm an Alien in *Deutschland*

Erhabor S. Idemudia
Klaus Boehnke

I'm an Alien in *Deutschland*

A Quantitative Mental Health Case Study of African Immigrants in Germany

With an epilogue by John W. Berry

PETER LANG
Frankfurt am Main · Berlin · Bern · Bruxelles · New York · Oxford · Wien

Bibliographic Information published by the Deutsche Nationalbibliothek
The Deutsche Nationalbibliothek lists this publication in the Deutsche Nationalbibliografie; detailed bibliographic data is available in the internet at http://dnb.d-nb.de.

This book was published with financial support from the Alexander von Humboldt-Foundation.

Cover Design:
Olaf Glöckler, Atelier Platen, Friedberg

ISBN 978-3-631-59975-4

www.peterlang.de

Foreword

The aim of this study is to describe the vagaries associated with globalization and international migration among Africans and account empirically and from a psychological perspective, the responses of Africans in novel cultural environments in Germany, the core assumption being that culture contact is inherently stressful. Running in tandem to this is providing empirical evidence that looks at how culture-induced stress is related to psychopathology.

The empirical material for the present study was gathered by the first author as an Alexander van Humboldt Fellow (AvH) at Jacobs University Bremen (formerly known as the International University Bremen (IU^B).

The authors are indebted to the ministries of the justice or interior of several German states (details are given in the book) for allowing them access to prisons under their administration.

They are yet more indebted to the participants of their study, who agreed to participate, often against major reservations.

Last but not least they are indebted to Rena Dickel and Bianca Bergmann, Team Assistants at Jacobs University Bremen for giving the book manuscript a thorough proofreading.

Readers should note that the present report is not meant to address legal specifics of African migrants in current-day Germany, nor does it offer a comprehensive review of all available literature of African migration in the 21st century. What it sets out to offer is material on the psychosocial wellbeing of African immigrants to Germany, obtained from a snowball sample of Africans living in Germany, with a certain focus on a comparison of detained immigrants with immigrants living in Germany 'freely,' under various legal circumstances.

Its primary audience is not so much German academia or other experts on Germany as a migration destination, but much more so the international reader lacking insight into the situation of African immigrants to a country in Europe without strong traditional ties to the African continent. In that way the study can be characterized as a—largely quantitative—case study of the psychosocial wellbeing of Africans in a Diaspora setting.

Table of Content

1. Introduction: Rational and Background

There is a long history of Africans migrating to other lands including Germany and other European Countries. According to Opitz, Oguntoye, and Schultz (1992), there is no precise method of determining when the first Africans came to Germany. However, there are accounts of paintings from the 12th Century that depict Africans living in Germany. Until well into the 19th Century, German contacts with Africa were restricted to trade relations which centered around gold, ivory, spices, and other raw materials. Later, human beings were also shipped to Europe in increasing numbers as "tokens"—traded or taken as security for contractual agreements. According to historian Joseph Ki-Zerbo (2003) humans were carried away primarily to prove that the Europeans had really been to Africa and to satisfy the curiosity of compatriots who wanted to see what Black people looked like. One major unique account from the eighteenth century period of possibly the first African was cited in Opitz, et al. of a Ghanaian by the name of A.W. Amo, who was brought to Germany in 1703 as a present to Count Anton Ulrich von Wolfenbüttel by the Dutch West India Company, one of the biggest slave trading enterprises of the time. The count and his son assumed sponsorship of Amo and sent him to the University of Halle, which at that time was bestowed with great fame by a faculty that included a number of important figures of the Enlightenment. Amo later became a lecturer, writer, philosopher, and was appointed by Friedrich Wilhelm I as a Member of State Council of the Prussian crown at the court in Berlin. As a philosopher, he became one of the most important exponents of Christian von Wolff's philosophy, and as a follower of John Locke's and Descartes' mechanical philosophy, he was prominent in the fight against the early Lutheran and pietistic clerics. His first scholarly work concerned the rights of the Moors in Europe and was published in 1729 under the Latin title "De jure mauro in Europa", but later seemingly was lost.

In the latter part of the 20th century and into the 21st century, many Africans migrated to Europe and the United States for educational pursuits while others travel to other countries, which they perceive as affluent for leisure, vacation, to work and even to emigrate. Today's world has been referred to as a 'global village' which is why people travel from one continent to another in few hours or even minutes and reasons for such migratory movement have been attributed to political, social, psychological, and economic factors.

What is worrisome and which is the bane of this study is not that Africans travel to other countries but the current trend and manner of the travel is unprecedented. Everyday, headlines on African migrants 'screams' on the many front pages of international and local electronic outlets and newsprints. Two illustrations are to be found below and on the next page, which allow an insight into headlines appearing around the turn of the millennium (Box 1, taken from taken from Sorious Samura's CNN documentary film *Exodus from Africa*, aired in Summer 2001), and headlines appearing in 2005 (Box 2).

Box 1

- 25,000 Congolese sought asylum in France between 1990/1999
- 500,000 immigrants entered Europe illegally in the year 2000
- Spain alone arrested 10,000 illegal immigrants in the year 2000
- 39,000 immigrants deported from EU Countries in year 2000 alone
- 20,000 illegal immigrants in detention
- More than 5,000 illegal immigrants were deported from Spain alone in year 2001
- Common EU Policy on immigrants not expected before 2004
- 400,000 illegal immigrants smuggle into EU each year
- Spanish government spends $20 million on border security measures alone

Many African youths believe that to put an end to one's problems is to travel to Europe and the North Americas thinking that it is all bed of roses: lands flowing with milk and honey. So they travel in droves and in fact many even travel by unsafe means. Some trek through the valleys and shadows of death of the hot Sahara desert, trolleys, dinghies and cargo ships. Some even meet their premature death while trying to cross over borders. Those who succeed, on arrival find that the land that was supposed to flow with 'milk and honey' actually flow with racism, hardships, imprisonment, police harassments, daily apprehension of deportation, and other hosts of hostile life situations. Coping life styles for some are then channeled into drug trade (a common sight in many a German *Hauptbahnhof,* main train stations), prostitution, and domestic thefts, and as a result, find their homes in prisons, lockouts, asylums, and mental institutions while some engage in petty and menial jobs such as dish washing in restaurants, corpse cleaning, etc. It is not uncommon to find university graduates washing dishes in restaurants, cleaning the streets, and engaging in jobs that are menial to 'keep body and soul together'. The consequences being psychological difficulties necessitated by settling in a new country, the frustrations and loneliness induced by racism, police harassments, and the inevitable clash of values which inevitably have implications for mental health and wellbeing. For some with strong resilience to stress the consequences may be in the long term while for those with weak resilience to stress, the consequences may be immediate.

Box 2

- African migrants storm razor-wire border, Deccan Herald, India, October 5, 2005
- Hundreds of Migrants charge Spain's African border, Reuters-UK, United Kingdom, October 5, 2005
- Africa at the ramparts of Fortress Europe, Spiegel Online, Germany, October 6, 2005
- African migrants risk all in 'do or die' odyssey, San Diego Union Tribune, United States, October 6, 2005
- Spanish amnesty worsened immigrant problem, Germany, Reuters-UK, United Kingdom, October 9, 2005
- Spain to begin expelling African migrants, Guardian Unlimited, United Kingdom, October 5, 2005
- Immigration on EU agenda, EU Politix.com, Belgium, October 11, 2005
- African Union worried over migrants, CNN International, October 12, 2005.
- Morocco flies hundreds of African migrants' home, Globe and Mail, Canada, October 12, 2005
- Morocco deports migrants, BBC News, United Kingdom, October 14, 2005
- African migrants in Sahara lose hope, Middle East Online, United Kingdom, October14, 2005

There is no doubt that moving from one society to another can cause emotional difficulties because migrants pass from one set of cultural values to another. Immigrants to other countries bring with them psychological responses to difficulties of their community. Different migrating populations have diverse resources and different abilities to cope with the stresses encountered. Immigrant groups are subject to discrimination in housing, employment, in education services and in everyday interpersonal relations. Also, in virtually all EU countries, housing of ethnic minorities indicates that they occupy the transitional zones of town areas, which are falling into disrepair and scheduled for eventual demolition in accommodation, which has rudimentary sanitation and cooking facilities (Littlewood & Lipsedge, 1989). In this context numerous questions arise that can loosely be taken as research questions pursued in the empirical study reported in the current volume, should though not be mistaken as being put to a full test: (1) How do the experience of racism and other difficulties affect the psychological adjustment of African minority groups in Germany? (2) What nature of mental problems do African migrants in Germany suffer from? (3) Is migration always followed by emotional difficulties? (4) Are difficulties related to the stresses of migration itself? (5) Is it possible that African migrant groups have high rates of some types or general psychopathology?[1] (6) What impact does coming to Germany have on their mental health? (7) What are the cross-cultural impacts on health of African Immigrants in Germany? (8) What value orientations and stereotypes do African immigrants have vis-à-vis German citizens? (9) How do these orientations and stereotypes affect them?

Unfortunately, there are no 'hard' data on life satisfaction and general wellbeing of African migrants and particularly that of those living in Germany. Although there is fair amount of 'hard' data on such questions as social values and stereotypes, almost no such data are available for African migrants in Germany generally. Not a single study has, as far as the authors know, emphasized the role of mental and emotional health of African migrants. It is in this light therefore, that this book focuses on African migrants living in Germany from a psychological perspective by documenting the nature and extent of mental difficulties suffered by Africans living in Germany.

The overall objectives of the present study can be described as follows:

- Exploring the psychological and social profiles of African men and women living in Germany;

---

1 A study of different ethnic groups in Birmingham showed in fact that the pattern of crime was similar to that found in mental illness when compared with the general population (Lambert, 1971).

- Understanding their emotional and mental status, including those serving jail terms or remanded in prisons, asylums, and lock-ups, and compare both populations;
- Understanding the interplay of demographics of African migrants and their mental health;
- Developing an action research scheme on mental and emotional aspects of African migrants in Germany including value orientations and stereotypes.

This study offers a bridge between studies in psychology, sociology, political and cultural studies. The multidisciplinary approach of it can claim to be quite unusual. The study, thus, is designed to aid correcting the inadequacies of mass exodus from African countries to other countries in Europe and America. The implicit aim of the book therefore is to help African migrants, particularly the youths, understand the 'troubles' of migration and its effects on wellbeing.

2 Migration Patterns in Africa—Political, Social and Economic Factors

As Adepoju (1992) ascertains, the history of African migration is as old as the history of the continent. People moved for political, economic, religious and security reasons. Also migration in Africa has been deeply affected by the colonial experiences, which in turn affected economic, social, cultural, political and demographic development. In Africa today, with a few exceptions, migration is based on colonial ties. For example, many English-speaking African migrants would rather migrate to the United Kingdom or even the United States whereas French-speaking Africans would prefer going to France and French-speaking countries.

However, the reason for the current cross-border movement which has led to an increase in the number of people moving from one country and continent to another rests squarely on globalization—largely an acronym for liberalization of international trade and the revolution in communication. Globalization is arguably one of the most important factors generating increased levels of international migration. For Africans, other factors for migration include economic and political development failures.

2.1 Globalization

Trade liberalization, according to Chimanikire (2002), has placed developing economies under economic pressures, often generating increased unemployment, reduced social spending and a decline in living standards. According to Boswell and Crisps (2004), such pressures no doubt generate political insecurity by creating grievances over limited or inequitably distributed resources, or frustration at the declining capacity of states to provide socio-economic security. Globalization, they say, has not only increased 'push factors' inducing emigration, but has expanded possibilities for the flow of information, communication and movement between states and also increased the demand for both high and low skilled workers. In fact, the media have described cross-border international migration as 'regionalization and globalization' of migration, and today international cross-border migrations have reached the top of the international agenda (Boswell & Crisp 2004).

Obviously, however, migrant flows are always from the poorest countries with a low probability of employment towards less poor and more dynamic countries where there is an opportunity to find some sort of job.

International migration according to Martin (2002) is usually a major individual or family decision that is carefully considered and has two broad categories: those who migrate to another country for primarily economic reasons, and those who move primarily for non-economic reasons. The factors that encourage a migrant to actually move, Martin grouped into three categories: demand-pull (reasons that draw people to particular destinations, such as the US, Canada, or Australia), supply-push (circumstances in the home environment that make a person think about leaving his normal place of abode for another part of the same country, neighboring countries, or to further distant countries) and network factors (e.g., family ties). Chimanikire (2002) has also described these categories as economic (employment, study, retirement), social (family or ethnic reasons, marriage unification) and political (refugees, persecution of war, famine, mass expulsion, and general political and economic disorder or environmental crises). Economic migrants will move due to the demand-pull factor as guest workers recruitment, while non-economic are likely to be motivated to cross borders to join family members, while others migrate because they hear or have been told about work and good conditions in abroad (network factors).

From early on, but all the time more since the end of the Cold War, the increased scale of international migration has been profoundly troubling to many receiving countries. According to Boswell and Crisp (2004), while the industrialized countries derive many benefits from immigration, there remains considerable public and political resistance to any liberalization of migration and asylum policy. This resistance they state is linked to a range of popular concerns about the allegedly negative impact of immigration and refugee flows on employment, welfare systems, national security and identity. As such fears, they claim, are unfounded, there indeed is a strong economic and demographic case for loosening restrictions on migration, government and opposition parties continue to mobilize electoral support through promises to obstruct, deter, or limit the arrival of foreign nationals into Europe and in Germany in particular.

However, the contradiction between the economic case for liberalization and the political pressures for closure has contributed to a number of negative and for the most part unintended consequences. According to Boswell and Crisp (2004), the consequences include use of illegal routes by migrants which has significantly increased human trafficking and smuggling networks, undermining of international refugee protection regime because those that are desperately in need of asylum cannot have it because the system has been abused by some migrants claiming asylum, and—on the other end of the spectrum, so-to-speak—the encouragement of high-skilled migration which no doubt is exacerbating the "brain-drain" problem in low-income countries, thereby further impeding their development.

Also, there are economic and political development failures in Africa. Most African immigrants are responding to push factors at home, namely economic development failures. In Europe, especially, many of these migrants are doing lower-skilled jobs despite the fact that they constitute people with very high education in their home countries. It is not uncommon to see an African graduate of accounting cleaning the streets of London, Paris, or Frankfurt.

2.2 Instability and Political Turmoil

Another strong motivation for Africans migrating to other countries comes about as a result of political turmoil in their countries, which in turn is linked to the political instability and failure of economic development. In many African countries, corruption is wide-spread, which is the bane of poverty within a rapid population growth, disease and illiteracy, and all these produce a volatile environment resulting in wars and famine, civil strife, riots and other forms of political violence almost inadvertently leading to the displacement of people as migrants, refugees or asylees.

Political instability due to greed by African leaders (take the case of Zimbabwe) has also been known to exacerbate the economic crisis in many African countries. Two thirds of Zimbabweans, for example, have fled their country. Severe political problems are also known to dominate the situation in Sudan and the Democratic Republic of Congo/Rwanda. According to Chimanikire (2004), it can be pointed out that over the last 40 years nearly 20 African countries [or about 40 % of Sub-Saharan Africa (SSA)] have experienced at least one period of civil war and it is estimated that 20 % of SSA's population now live in countries which are formally at war or where low-intensity conflict has become endemic. This gloomy and negative state in Africa has led many to describe Africa as a doomed and 'Dark Continent.'

In conclusion, it is important to know that the globalization of economies, lack of development and political instability in many African countries and to some extent immigration policies of some industrialized nations are responsible for Africans migrating to neighboring and other countries.

3. Theoretical Perspectives

There is no single, welldeveloped theory of international migration. Quite a number of models used to explain international migration have been proposed by economists, political scientists, and sociologists. These are not in the center of our interest. However, there are theoretical perspectives guarded by psychosocial model rather than economic or political macro-concerns, which highlight the significance of life changes and the appraisal of these changes during migration. According to Ward, Bochner, and Furnham (2001), the stress-coping framework assumes that the experience of intercultural contact and change occurs in a socio-political and economic context and is influenced by the characteristics of the migrant's society of origin and the society of settlement. The changes associated with these types of contact are viewed as precipitating stress, resulting in affective, behavioral and cognitive coping responses. Therefore, both stress and coping are mediated by characteristics of the individual and characteristics of the situation, and in turn, affect adjustive outcomes.

Berry (1997) considers the acculturative experience as a major life event that is characterized by stress, demands cognitive appraisal of the situation, and requires coping strategies. These processes and their psychological outcomes are likely to be influenced by both societal composition and individual level variables. Society of origin, group acculturation, and society of settlement, and various individual variables are strong factors affecting acculturation experience and level of stress.

Another major theoretical account on why social contact between culturally disparate individuals is difficult and often stressful is the similarity-attraction hypothesis (Byrne, 1969). This theoretical account predicts that individuals are more likely to seek out, enjoy, understand, want to work and play with, trust, believe, vote for, and generally prefer people with whom they share salient characteristics. These include interests, values, religion, group affiliation, skills, physical attributes, age, language, and all the other aspects on which human beings can differ (or be similar). And, since cultural identification by definition categorizes people according to the idiosyncratic characteristics, which distinguish them from other groups, it follows that cross-cultural interactions occur between individuals who are likely to be dissimilar on at least some of these salient dimensions. A close analogy would be that societies could in principle be located on a continuum of how close or distant they are with respect to their sociocultural features (Babiker, Cox &

Miller, 1980). According to Ward, Bochner, and Furnham (2001) the culture-distance hypothesis predicts that the greater the cultural gap between people in contact, the more difficulties they will experience.

Abrams and Hogg (1990) have also proposed that cross-cultural interaction is inherently difficult because of the process of social categorization, a term used to refer to the tendency of individuals to classify others as members of a group, in particular whether they belong to their own, in-group, or to some other, out-group. This form of categorization of people has consequences for how people so categorized are perceived and treated, the in-group usually (Tajfel, 1970, 1981), but not always (e.g. Bochner & Cairns, 1976) being given preference. The process of stereotyping (Katz & Braly, 1933; Lippmann, 1922) also contributes to the dynamics of intercultural contact, in attributing to individuals the traits that allegedly characterize the group that the target person has been assigned to by the perceiver.

Primary socialization, as theorized several decades ago (Deaux, 1976), is the process through which persons acquire a set of core values early in their lives, which they come to regard as reflecting reality and, therefore, as absolutely true, and which, for a variety of reasons, are fairly resistant to change. And again by definition, different cultures may and do provide idiosyncratic primary socializing influences. This may result in belief systems that are not universally shared and values that are diametrically opposed but greatly cherished by their respective groups. When members of two such groups come into contact, the potential for conflicts are obvious (Ward, Bochner, and Furnham, 2001).

Another source of inter-cultural conflict has been termed ‘cultural syndromes’ (Triandis, 1990). Cultural syndromes refer to patterns of attitudes, beliefs, norms and behaviors that can be used to contrast groups of cultures. Triandis (1990) identified three major cultural syndromes that are relevant to the analysis of ethnocentrism: cultural complexity, tight versus loose cultures, and individualism-collectivism. He also considered the implications of theses syndromes for effective intercultural relations. For example, people from tight cultures prefer certainty and security. Because they highly value predictability, they are likely to reject people from loose cultures, perceiving them as unreliable and undisciplined. People from complex cultures pay attention to time, while people from less complex cultures tend to ignore time. This difference has an almost proverbial relevance for relations between Africans and Germans.

The theme of this book therefore follows the argument that migrants (in this case Africans) will no doubt have difficulties living in a foreign land like Germany. Points of difficulties will arise due to barriers inherent in the host country and, in addition, to language difficulties (as most Africans only learn the German language after their arrival in Germany or don't bother at all). Language problems can create barriers in effective communication; sow the seed of misunderstanding, friction and hostility and consequently racial prejudice. Some researchers (Tanaka, Takai, Kohyama, & Fujihara, 1994; Ward & Searle, 1991) have argued that attitudes held by members of the dominant culture strongly influence patterns of immigrant's adaptation. In fact, according to Fernando (1993), racism is the most serious risk factor for immigrants. Also, a few studies (Ataca, 1996; Furnham & Shiekh, 1993) have looked into the correlates of perceived discriminations or prejudice and findings have revealed a uniform negative association between perceptions of racism and psychological wellbeing. It is important to note that theory and research on values and attitudes (perceptions) have a place in the cognitive-based social identification theories. According to Ward, Bochner, and Furnham (2001) values as evaluative beliefs are cognitive constructs intimately tied to self-definition and cultural identity, and can significantly be affected by intercultural contact. It is within this framework that this book therefore investigates the psychology of African migrants in Germany. Migrants here refer to Africans living in Germany. They include legal and illegal residents. No temporary visitors were interviewed for this study. Some illegal residents had filed for political asylum and had not been granted it. The mean length of stay/residence in Germany is 7 ½ years with a high standard deviation of 4 ½ years.

3.1 Mental Health

According to Opitz, Oguntoye, and Schultz (1992) the unification of the two Germanies has not only brought severe economic problems but also has changed the political and social climate in both the East and the West. It is significant that with the fall of the Wall, white Germans from the German Democratic Republic (GDR) were greeted sympathetically by West Germans, while Black Germans, immigrants, and refugees have been confronted with increasingly open racism. The new immigration laws, *Ausländergesetze*, of the united Federal Republic of Germany, which was drafted long before unification, was passed in 1990 and became valid on January 1, 1991. It contains, among other points, severely intensified restrictions on immigration and residence permits; it also makes civil servants liable for reporting on the living and working condition and conduct of immigrants. This information can be used as grounds for deportation.

Within a year of German unification, the European Union—as a meant-to-be political union—came to force in 1992. Since then, Europe is seen by many as having developed into an economic and political bulwark against the rest of the world, above all against the countries and peoples of what used to be called the Third World in Cold War times. Already today, migratory movements and immigration are being controlled, curtailed, and/or stopped altogether through international agreements (e.g., the Schengen Agreement of 1989). As a result, Europe has been dubbed by the media as the "fortress Europe."

Access to health and wellbeing are factors that are also strongly related to discrimination among African migrants in Germany (Idemudia, 2005). Gorman, Brough, and Ramirez (2003), have also claimed that people with a non–English-speaking background (NESB) are disadvantaged in terms of access and quality of service in Australian monocultural Anglo-Celtic health setting, a supposedly officially acknowledged multicultural society. Logiudice, Hassett, Cook, Flicker, & Ames (2001) have earlier also made similar observation that due to an absence of sensitivity and understanding, young people and all culturally and linguistically diverse (CALD) clients do not have sufficient access to mental health services, and have claimed that such clients are at risk of poor or even destructive experiences when they do access them (Blackford, Street, & Parsons, 1997; Comino, Silove, Manicavasagar, Harris, & Harris, 2001).

3.2 Gender Differences

It is, however, important to note that migration and health can be related positively or negatively in a number of ways. Literature to date has shown that the relationship can be controversial. There is no doubt that moving from one society to another can cause emotional difficulties. Different migrating populations have diverse resources and different abilities to cope with the stresses encountered. It is common-place that immigrant groups are subject to discrimination in housing, employment, in education services and in everyday interpersonal relations (see, e.g., Littlewood & Lipsedge, 1989),

Discrimination, particularly racial discrimination has been known to exacerbate psychological dysfunctions among migrants in Europe (Idemudia & Boehnke, 2005; 2006; Idemudia, 2006). Fernando (1993) sees racism as the most serious risk factor for immigrants. Other researchers (Vega, Gil, Warheit, Zimmerman, & Apospori, 1993; Ward & Chang, 1997) have also found negative correlates of perceived discriminations or prejudice and psychological wellbeing.

According to Hutchinson and Haasen (2004), there is increased risk of schizophrenia for non-white migrants in Europe, with Africans and individuals from the Caribbean being especially vulnerable in the United Kingdom; and Turkish migrants in Germany. The same type of increased risk has also been found among Caribbean, East and West African migrants to the Netherlands. Social inequalities, family fragmentation and migratory stress have been the main hypothesis proposed for the vulnerabilities and increased rates. How this increased risk for migrants affect gender is not known.

Explanations of mental health among migrant population tend to be anchored on the so-called migration-morbidity hypothesis (Klimidis & Minas, 1995) advanced to suggest a link between the prevalence of psychiatric disorder and migrant status. Although, Gorman, Brough and Ramirez (2003), has viewed the hypothesis as too simplistic because of the complex nature of psychiatric morbidity and migrant status which involves risk factors such as socioeconomic status, pre-migration stresses and gender of migrant.

Unfortunately, risk factors for gender and wellbeing of African migrants are essentially unknown. According to Marshall (1994), gender refers to socially constructed aspects of differences between men and women. Since its introduction as a social concept it has been extended to refer not only to individual identity and personality but also, the symbolic level, to cultural ideas and stereotypes of masculinity and femininity.

However, there is a growing interest among social science researchers in the comparative male-female vulnerability to several stressful life circumstances that have been implied in the development of psychopathology. Three major explanations have been suggested: the differential vulnerability hypothesis, the differential exposure hypothesis, and social role theory. The differential vulnerability hypothesis assumes that given exposure to similar life stresses and strains, women are more likely than men to manifest symptoms of psychopathology. The hypothesis focuses on both contextual factors and features of feminine socialization that may render women more inclined than men to react to life difficulties with feelings of self-blame and a sense of helplessness and hopelessness (Brown & Harris, 1978; Makosky, 1982). The hypothesis of differential exposure focuses on the role that various work-related strains play in contributing to excessive levels of psychopathology among women, in general, and married women in particular (Aneshensel, Frerichs & Clark 1981, Cleary and Mechanic, 1983). However, the work of Makosky (1980, 1982) and Greywolf, Ashlay, and Reese (1982) raises questions as to whether such strains are the most salient risk factors for depression in the lives of women. These authors emphasize the etiological significance of a very different set of life strains such as the absence of a spouse, social isolation, chronic poverty, and poor health, all of which involve major resource deficits that have been linked to depression (Warheit, 1975).

Although the social-role theory is frequently referred to as a sex-role theory (e.g. Rosenfield, 1980), the explanatory framework developed by Gove and Tudor (1973) clearly invokes gender-specific roles, husband/wife, father/mother, worker/housewife, rather than the global male and female sex roles to account for gender differences in mental illness. Gove (1972) specifically claimed that it is the roles that women occupy, rather than some characteristics of women's generalized sex role, which make women more susceptible to mental illness. A key explanatory element in this orientation in the purported greater stress placed on married women, as compared with that placed on married men or the unmarried of both sexes, by extensive familial role demands. However, studies based on social role theory have shown mixed results. Radloff (1978) reports that marital status, employment status, and sex interact in their relationship to mental illness, but conclude that these social roles are inadequate to account for sex differences in mental illness. Fox (1980) presented results of three different national studies of untreated mental illness, which indicate that women are more likely to be mentally ill than men regardless of marital status. These findings therefore lead to the conclusion that the theory at least to some degree lacks internal validity.

However, Weissman and Klerman (1977) maintain that there is strong evidence that social role contributes to the vulnerability of women to mental illness. One way in which it might, they hypothesize, is in the discrimination against women inherent in their disadvantaged social status. Real social discrimination makes it difficult for women to achieve mastery by direct action and self assertion, and this leads to legal and economic helplessness, dependency on others, low self-esteem, low aspirations, and ultimately mental illness. Beck and Greenberg (1974) also suggested that the problems which typically trigger depression may be 'sex-typed', point out that the absence of power to control one's own life is more commonly experienced by women than by men. Seligman (1975) believes that people are more likely to become depressed when they have learned that their actions will have no effect. The cause of depression is learned helplessness, or the belief that action is futile. Radloff and Monroe (1978) maintain that women learn helplessness from the feminine stereotype, the treatment of female children, the status of women in political and economic institutions, and the experience of being dominated at home.

Despite the plausibility of these hypotheses, few studies have investigated whether women are more vulnerable to psychopathology than men, given exposure to similar life difficulties and strains. Studies that do address this question have produced mixed results, some suggesting a greater female vulnerability to depression in the face of interpersonal problems and difficulties (Kessler & McLeod, 1984; Newmann, 1982); others pointing to a greater male vulnerability to depression in relation to problems with the breadwinner role, including job stresses and strains (Radloff & Rae, 1981), yet other studies pointing to income losses (Kessler & McLeod, 1984). Thus, while these findings suggest some support for the hypothesis that women may be more vulnerable than men to symptoms of mental illness, such vulnerability appears to be largely specific to interpersonal strains.

From the above account, it is obvious that there is paucity of research on gender differences to psychopathology among migrants and as such a systematic pattern of observation on the excess of symptomatology in males or females is yet to emerge. In Africa, women are not treated as equals by males. The relevance and importance is all too obvious in cultural issues. Men are seen as head of houscholds. These cultural and social beliefs are somewhat different in the western world. In Germany, women are equal to men in the legal sense and also with regard to some more symbolic domains of life, not though economically. In the year 2000 women in West Germany earned about 78 % of what men earned on average, while in East Germany, with its higher gender equality of the job market, women earned 87 % of what men earned (Frank-Bosch, 2002). Given stressful situations in Europe, who would report more symptoms: males or females? This study is an attempt to contribute to the male-female debate on vulnerability to psychopathology and also to try and address the paucity of data, especially quantitative material on gender and mental health which would help provide empirical data of mental health of African migrants in a European country (Germany). The general scenario is that when families want to migrate from Africa, the men leave first and when life conditions have improved, the man then asks the wife or girlfriend to join him. With this scenario, the men have the first opportunity to experience all the hardships that comes with migration. With this understanding therefore, men are likely more than women to report negative problems making them *ceteris paribus*, to report more symptoms of psychological dysfunctions.

3.3. Research Question

As mentioned in the foreword to the current volume and adding to the description of the general scope of our research (Chapter 1), we should once again stress that our study does not set out to test specific hypotheses but sees itself as a quantitative case study of African migrants to Germany. For that population the interrelation of acculturative stress, personal values, and mental health is explored with a side-focus on a cross-gender comparison and a comparison of incarcerated and "free" individuals. Although there are no specific hypotheses tested in the current study, our research nevertheless is based on general assumptions. We expect self-reported acculturative stress being substantively related to psychopathology. We expect the two genders and individuals from the two "life-contexts" (prison and "freedom") to differ in their mental health status. Expectations with regard to gender have been outlined above; we expect men to exhibit a poorer mental health status. With regard to "life-context," we expect prison inmates to have a poorer mental health status than respondents from the general population, without, though, being able to say whether this reflects a selection phenomenon (people with a poorer mental health more likely to be incarcerated), or a socialization phenomenon (imprisonment weakening mental health). As for values, we see them as a possible moderator between acculturative stress and mental health: Acculturative stress is likely to be easier to bear, for example, for people who seek stimulation in life than for people who cherish security. Furthermore, Africans whose value preference profile deviates from the typical profile of Germans will experience acculturative stress more immediately than Africans whose values resemble those of average Germans more closely. The former group can be assumed to be more prone to experience mental health problems.

4. Methodology

The study was in principle a survey study, amended with a one-time focus group discussion for purposes of data triangulation.

The focus group discussion, in which ten African migrants participated, took place in a meeting center of Nigerians in central Bremen. During the focus group discussion participants were asked to also provide thorough life stories that served as points of departure of the discussion, and offered insights into migration patterns and networks, as well as problems encountered in Germany. Focus group discussion participants also responded to a mini-questionnaire aimed at acquiring evidence on the interrelation between various demographic variables (including reasons for emigration from their country) and problems encountered in Germany. Material from the focus group interviews is not reported in detail in the present volume, but is used as background material for interpretations offered to explain findings reported in the later sections of the book.

Before we proceed to describing in detail the sample of African migrants in Germany to which the present research pertains, a more in-depth look at some parameters of modern-day Germany seems in place. Some of the information given in the subsequent section relies heavily on material published in the "Germany: Facts and Figures" segment of the *about.com* website.

4.1 Setting: Germany

Although Germany is not one of the classical immigration countries (e.g., United States of America, Canada, Australia, Israel, or New Zealand), and is also a country without strong colonial ties in Africa, an increasing presence of African immigrants has become obvious. Germany lost its African colonies after World War I in the Treaty of Versailles. Before World War I Germany held colonies in South-West Africa, now Namibia and a small part of Botswana, West Africa, now Cameroon and Togo, and East Africa, now part of Tanzania, Rwanda, Burundi, and a small part of Kenya and of Mozambique.

Today, Germany is a country with an immigrant population of over 10 million people, a figure including recent naturalizations, thereby taking Rank 3 in the World after the US (35.4 million) and Russia (12.1 million)[2].

Germany has a total population of 82.5 million (World Factbook, 2009). Of this figure, 91.5 % are German nationals. Among the non-nationals Turks form the largest group (2.4 %), with immigrants from former Yugoslavia, Italians, Poles, and Greeks forming the next largest groups. The relatively largest non-European groups come from the US, Vietnam, and China. Altogether about 270,000 African nationals lived in Germany in 2007.[3] Their average age was 32.5, and their average length of stay in Germany was 11 ½ years. Moroccans form the largest African group of non-German nationals (an estimated 70,000 in 2006). The largest groups of sub-Saharan nationals living in Germany come from Ghana (app. 20,500), Nigeria (app. 16,000), and Ethiopia (app. 10,000)[4].

Less than 100,000 non-German nationals obtained German citizenship through naturalization in 2008, among them about 9.600 Africans, with about 40 % of them from sub-Saharan Africa.[5]

The Federal Republic of Germany (*Bundesrepublik Deutschland*), bordering the Baltic and the North Sea, is in a way Europe's dominant country, both in economic power and population (World Factbook, 2009). Located approximately in the centre of Europe, Germany is comparable in size to Zimbabwe and the Republic of Congo (Brazzaville). The country shares common borders with Denmark, Poland, the Czech Republic, Austria, Switzerland, France, Luxembourg, Belgium, and the Netherlands.

Today Germany is the European Union's most populous nation. However, Germany as a unified nation is much newer than most of its European neighbors. Germany was founded as a unified nation and had her independence on January 18, 1871 under the leadership of Chancellor Otto von Bismarck, after Prussia (*Preußen*) had conquered most of German-speaking Europe. Prior to that, "Germany" had been a loose association of 39 German

---

2 http://www.un.org/esa/population/publications/2006Migration_Chart/Migration2006.pdf

3 http://www.destatis.de/jetspeed/portal/cms/Sites/destatis/SharedContent/Oeffentlich/AI/IC/Publikationen/ Jahrbuch/Bevoelkerung,property=file.pdf

4 http://de.statista.com/statistik/daten/studie/1221/umfrage/anzahl-der-auslaender-in-deutschland-nach-herkunftsland/

5 https://www-ec.destatis.de/csp/shop/sfg/bpm.html.cms.cBroker.cls?cmspath=struktur,vollanzeige.csp&ID= 1024112

states known as the German League (*Deutscher Bund*). The German Empire reached its zenith under Emperor (*Kaiser*) Wilhelm II just prior to the start

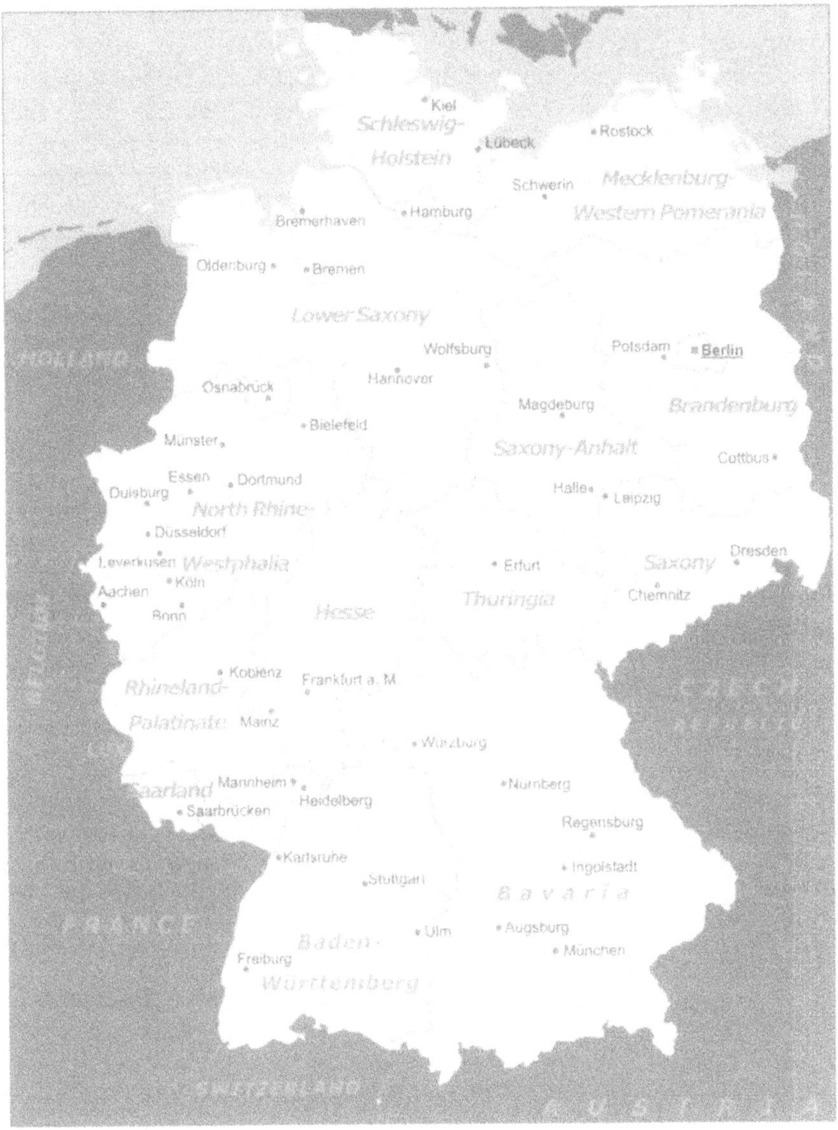

Figure 1: *Political Map of Germany*

of World War I in 1914. After the end of WW I in 1918, Germany attempted to become a democratic republic in 1919, but the so-called Weimar Republic proved to be only a short-lived prelude to the rise of Adolf Hitler and the dictatorial "Third Reich" of the Nazis. Following World War II in 1945, the country was divided into four zones of occupation (UK, US, USSR, and later, France). The western part of the country became the Federal Republic of Germany (FRG, or West Germany), proclaimed May 23, 1949, and included the former UK, US, and French zones. Its eastern part, the German Democratic Republic (GDR, or East Germany) was proclaimed October 7, 1949, and included the former Soviet zone. Unification of West Germany and East Germany took place October 3, 1990, and all four-power rights formally relinquished 15 March 1991.

After the Second World War, one man often gets most of the credit for creating today's democratic Federal Republic of Germany. In 1949, Christian Democrat Konrad Adenauer became the new Germany's first chancellor, sometimes labeled the "George Washington" of West Germany[6], a questionable honor, as this label had been used by the British politician Lloyd George for Adolf Hitler some years before (von Nostitz, 1967). That same year also saw the birth of communist East Germany (*Deutsche Demokratische Republik*) in the former Soviet Occupation Zone, ruled by the Socialist Unity Party (*Sozialistische Einheitspartei Deutschlands*) for 39 ½ years. For the next forty years, Germany's people and its history would be divided into an eastern and a western part. But it was not until August 1961 that a wall physically split the two Germanys. The Berlin Wall (*Mauer*) and the barbed wire fence that lined the entire border between East and West Germany became a major symbol of the Cold War. By the time the Wall fell in November 1989, Germans had lived two separate national lives for four decades. Many Germans, including West German then-Chancellor Helmut Kohl, underestimated the difficulties of reunifying people that had been divided and living under very different conditions for 40 years. Even today, some two decades after the Wall's collapse, true unification is still a goal in many societal spheres, but in hindsight Germany had probably no realistic choice other than unification, once the barrier of the Wall was gone.

Germany's constitution (*Grundgesetz*, Basic Law) of May 23, 1949 became unified Germany's constitution on October 3, 1990 (now a national holiday, *Tag der Deutschen Einheit*). There are two federal legislative bodies. The *Bundestag* is Germany's House of Representatives or lower house. Its mem-

---

6 http://german.about.com/b/2003/11/16/konrad-adenauer.htm

bers are elected to four-year terms in popular elections. The *Bundesrat* (Federal Council) is Germany's upper house. Its members are not elected but are the members of the federal state governments or their representatives. By law the upper house must approve any law that affects the *Länder*. The Federal President (*Bundespräsident*) is the titular head of state, but has no real political power. He/she holds office for a five-year term and can be re-elected only once. The current—recently reelected to a second term—Federal President is Horst Köhler. The Federal Chancellor (*Bundeskanzler*) is the German "premier" and political leader. He/she is elected by the Bundestag for a four-year term. The current federal chancellor is Angela Merkel, heading a grand coalition government formed by Christian and Social Democrats. The Federal Constitutional Court (*Bundesverfassungsgericht*) is the highest court of the land and the guardian of the Basic Law. There are lower federal and state courts. Germany has 16 federal states (*Länder*) with governmental powers similar to those of states in the US. West Germany had 11 Länder; the five so-called "new states" (*neue Länder*) of East Germany were reconstituted after unification. The GDR had 15 districts, each named for its capital city.

In 2008, religious groups in Germany included Roman Catholics (*katholisch*) 30.0 %; Protestants (*evangelisch*), 29.9 %; Muslims, 3.9 %; and people with other religious affiliations, 1.8 %. The remaining 34.1 % of the population have no religious affiliation[7], thereby making Germany one of the countries with the highest percentage of religiously non-affiliated inhabitants, many of them declared atheists (Zuckerman, 2007; Jagodzinski & Greeley, 1998). Since 2002, the monetary unit of Germany is the euro, which replaced the Deutsche Mark at that time.

With a per capita GDP around 35,000 US $ (PPP), Germany ranks somewhere between Ranks 14—in the World Bank[8] ranking—and 34—in the CIA World Factbook[9] ranking—in the world. It must be emphasized, however, that when looking at overall GDP (PPP) Germany takes Rank 5 after the United States, China, Japan, and India. The *World Factbook* summarizes the 2009 economic situation of Germany as follows: “The German economy—the fifth largest economy in the world in PPP terms and Europe's largest—began to contract in the second quarter of 2008 as the strong euro, high oil prices, tighter credit markets, and slowing growth abroad took their

---

7 http://www.fowid.de/

8 http://siteresources.worldbank.org/INTGLOMONREP2008/Resources/4737994-1207342962709/8944_Web_PDF.pdf

9 https://www.cia.gov/library/publications/the-world-factbook

toll on Germany's export-dependent economy. At 1.3 % in 2008, GDP growth is expected to be negative in 2009. Recent stimulus and lender relief efforts will make demands on Germany's federal budget and undercut plans to balance its budget by 2011. The reforms launched by the former government of Chancellor Gerhard Schröder, deemed necessary due to chronically high unemployment and low average growth, led to strong growth in 2007, while unemployment in 2008 fell below 8 %, a new post-reunification low. Germany's aging population, combined with high chronic unemployment, has pushed social security outlays to a level exceeding contributions, but higher government revenues from the cyclical upturn in 2006-07 and a 3 % rise in the value-added tax cut Germany's budget deficit to within the EU's 3 % debt limit in 2007. The current government of Chancellor Angela Merkel has initiated other reform measures, such as a gradual increase in the mandatory retirement age from 65 to 67 and measures to increase female participation in the labor market. The modernization and integration of the eastern German economy—where unemployment still exceeds 30 % in some municipalities—continues to be a costly long-term process, with annual transfers from west to east amounting to roughly $80 billion. While corporate restructuring and growing capital markets have set strong foundations to help Germany meet the longer-term challenges of European economic integration and globalization, Germany's export-oriented economy has proved a disadvantage in the context of weak global demand."

4.2 Design and Sampling

Our research project set out to study two groups of sub-Saharan African migrants to Germany, first, the general population of sub-Saharan Africans living in Germany, whether endowed with a legal residence permit status or not, and, second, incarcerated sub-Saharan Africans, who were at the time of the survey inmates of a German prison. The original aim of the research was to reach out to 300 African migrants. To reach this aim, about 600 questionnaire booklets were printed and distributed using a snowballing technique, encompassing in the following cities: Bremen, Hamburg, Bonn, Frankfurt am Main, Düsseldorf, Köln (Cologne), Bayreuth, Stuttgart, Koblenz, Neustadt an der Weinstraße in the State of Rhineland-Palatinate, Berlin, Hannover, and München (Munich). The return rate of questionnaires was, however, very low; only about 11 % of the questionnaires were returned. The main reason according to participants was that they were not sure if the first author was an agent of the German Government. Whether this response rate affects the quality of the findings, is extremely difficult to assess. Holbrook, Krosnick, and Pfent (2007) have shown that there is no systematic relationship between response rates and the size of bias encountered in surveys, but on the other hand, the selectivity of the present sample may mean that the sampled respondents are in general healthier from a psychopathology viewpoint than the average sub-Saharan African living in Germany. This guess cannot be refuted easily as participants of the general population segment of the study did after all volunteer to take part in an unusual study against the odds that one could have been suspicious vis-à-vis the intentions of the research. More than half of the respondents presumably did not have a legal residence status in Germany.

For the prison population, authorities in 12 German states were contacted for possible permission to solicit respondents from prisons under the jurisdiction of their state. Only Bavaria, Berlin, Bremen, Hessen, Mecklenburg-Western Pomerania, and Schleswig-Holstein responded positively, in principle, on the ministerial level. It usually took an average of about 2-3 months to get a response from the justice ministry and prison authorities. Many of the prison participants also were afraid of the motive of the study despite several clarifications made to them. In addition, few—if any—African inmates were available in prisons that gave permission at the time of the study. There also was a constant movement of prisoners around prisons in Germany.

Both among the general population and the prison population, study participants were requested to return the booklets by post in pre-paid envelopes that were also given out. This strategy was used to eliminate any possibility to identify respondents. For the prison population it was secured with the authorities that questionnaires would neither be censored nor copied. The authorities insisted, however, that outgoing letters would be opened for security reasons.

Altogether, data were collected from 85 African migrants living in Germany, 62 from the general population, 23 from the prison population.

4.3 Survey

As stated before, for the present study a survey was carried out among Africans living in Germany, using a structured questionnaire. The questionnaire contained several sections. Section A requested background (demographic) information on variables such as age, sex, educational qualification, migration variables like length of stay in Germany, and reasons for leaving home. It also asked for a brief statement on experiences in Germany and with the Germans in an open question. Section B contained the Minnesota Multiphasic Personality Inventory (MMPI), Section C contained the Migration Attitude Questionnaire (MAQ) developed for the study by the first author, and Section D contained a modified version of the Schwartz Value Survey (PVQ, Schwartz et al., 2001).

4.4 Instruments

4.4.1 Minnesota Multiphasic Personality Inventory-2 (MMPI-2)

The new Minnesota Multiphasic Personality Inventory-2 (Helmes & Reddon, 1993, Newmark & McCord, 1996) was used for the study. MMPI-2 is a re-standardized version of the original MMPI (Hathaway, 1960, Hathaway & McKinley, 1943). MMPI-2 contains, among other scales, 10 clinical scales, 3 validity scales and 15 content scales. This standardized personality test is the most extensively researched and widely used tool in the world. It has been translated to more than 100 languages (Myers, 1995) and, although it assesses psychological disorders rather than "normal" personality traits, its uses are extended to several areas. The Content Scales include: Anxiety (ANX), Fears (FRS), Obsessiveness (OBS), Depression (DEP), Health Concerns (HEA), Bizarre Mentation (BIZ), Anger (ANG), Cynicism (CYN), Antisocial Practices (ASP), Type A (TPA), Low Self-Esteem (LSE), Social Discomfort (SOD), Family Problems (FAM), Work Interference (WRK), Negative Treatment Indicators (TRY), L(ie) Scale, F Scale (a "fake bad" scale), and a K Scale to measure defensiveness tendencies. Scale scores are assessed in the form of so-called T scores.

In detail, the Content Scales are constructed as measuring the following:

1. Anxiety (ANX): A high score in ANX indicates general symptoms of anxiety including tension, somatic problems (such as heart pounding and shortness of breath), sleep difficulties, worries, and poor concentration.

2. Fears (FRS): A high score on FRS characterizes an individual with many specific fears, such as fear of high places, animals, fire, being indoors, etc.

3. Obsessiveness (OBS): Individuals with high scores on OBS have great difficulty making decisions and are likely to ruminate excessively about issues and problems. They are excessive worriers and frequently overwhelmed by their own thoughts.

4. Depression (DEP): High scores on this scale characterize significant depressive thoughts, such as apathy about life, feelings of hopelessness thoughts of suicide etc.

5. Health Concerns (HEA): Individuals with high scores on HEA report many physical symptoms across several body systems, such as gastrointestinal, neurological, cardiovascular, respiratory and other symptoms.

6. Bizarre Mentation (BIZ): Psychotic thought processes characterize individuals high on the BIZ scale. They may report peculiar thoughts, hallucination, and paranoid ideation (e.g., the belief that someone is trying to poison them).

7. Anger (ANG): High scores on the ANG scale suggest anger-control problems. These individuals report being irritable, impatient, hotheaded, annoyed, stubborn, and sometimes lose self-control.

8. Cynicism (CYN): Individuals who score high on CYN report misanthropic beliefs such as expecting negative motives behind the acts of others or holding negative attitudes toward those close to them.

9. Antisocial Practices (ASP): High score is ASP indicates behavior problems. Such individuals may report enjoying criminals' acts.

10. Type A (TPA): High scorers on TPA are hard driving, fast moving, individuals who frequently become impatient, irritable, and annoyed.

11. Low Self-Esteem (LSE): High scores on LSE characterize individuals with low opinions of themselves, such as believing that they are not liked by others and a burden to others.

12. Social Discomfort (SOD): Individuals with high scores in SOD are very uneasy around others, preferring to be by themselves. They see themselves as shy and disliked by others.

13. Family Problems (FAM): Considerable family discomfort, such as unpleasant and quarrelsome family members lacking love, or an unhappy marriage, lacking affection, are reported by high scores on FAM.

14. Work Interference (WRK): A high score on WRK is indicative of behaviors or attitudes such as low self-confidence, concentration difficulties, obsessiveness, tension and pressure, and decision-making problems which are likely to contribute to poor work performance.

15. Negative Treatment Indicators (TRY): High scores in TRY indicate individuals with negative attitudes towards doctors and mental health treatment. They do not believe anyone can understand or help them.

16. L Scale: High scores (T > 65) in the L scale indicate that the individual may not be honest in responding to the items in MMPI-2. T-scores between 55 and 65 demonstrate defensiveness, conventional and socially conforming behavior. These individuals appear to have little or no insight into motivation and over value their worth by utilizing repression and denial excessively. When the F and the K are also elevated the L scale may suggest full-blown clinical confusion that may be either organic or functional.

17. F Scale: individuals with F scores greater than 100 (variable response inconsistency) indicate random response or possibly "faking bad".

18 K Scale: High scores on the K scale indicate that the individual has taken the test more defensively or maintain appearance of adequacy than the average person. Low scores indicate true response set.

The MMPI-2 is answered 'Yes' or 'No'. Computation of scores for all measures was such that half-standard deviation above and below the mean was used to cut off low and high scorers. High scores on any psychological measures indicate a high report of psychological dysfunction.

Psychometric properties of the original MMPI-2 scales range from .89 (Depression), .89 (Health Concerns), .65 (Bizarre Mentation), .79 (Anger),

.78 (Low Self Esteem), .92 (Social Discomfort) to .86 (Family Problems), .85 (Work Interference) and .75 for Negative Treatment. Using samples of 1,425 subjects in Ibadan, Nigeria, Berner (1998) standardized the MMPI-2 content and validity scales among the Yoruba population. Validity coefficients (alpha coefficients) for all the scales used in this study ranged from .71 to .96, which demonstrates that the scales were valid for use. A pre-test of the scales was carried among 31 African migrants in Germany. Split-half reliability obtained for this sample ranged from .70 to .94 on the ten clinical scales used. This also indicates that the MMPI-2 was highly reliable for use among Africans in Germany.

Altogether, the MMPI-2 has about 560 items, a number difficult to handle in a non-clinical, non-student sample. "Only" 8 of the 10 clinical scales were used, but in spite of this shortening of the instrument, the questionnaire booklet came with almost 400 questions compressed into 10 pages. As a result, participants complained of the length and bulk of the booklet, most likely another reason for the low response rate.

4.4.2 Schwartz Value Survey (PVQ)

This measure is based on the theory of human values developed by Schwartz (1992). The approach defines values as desirable, transsituational goals, varying in importance, that serve as guiding principles in people's lives (Schwartz, 1992; cf. Kluckhohn, 1951; Rokeach, 1973). Values are cognitive representations of people's important goals or motivations, phrased in socially acceptable language useful for coordinating action. The primary content aspect that distinguishes among values is the type of motivational goal they express. Ten motivationally distinct types of values were derived from universal requirements of the human condition and validated in cross-cultural research (Schwartz, 1992, 1994; Schwartz & Sagiv, 1995). Table 1 lists these ten value types. Each type is defined in terms of its central goal (that is, the desired end state to which it is directed). Specific single values that primarily represent each type appear in parentheses following the definitions. A single value represents a value type when actions that express the value or lead to its attainment promote the central goal of the type.

In addition to identifying ten motivational types of values, the theory explicates a structural aspect of values, namely, the dynamic relations among them

(Schwartz, 1992). Actions in pursuit of any value have psychological, practical, and social consequences that may conflict or may be congruent with the pursuit of other values. For example, the pursuit of achievement values may conflict with the pursuit of benevolence values: seeking success for self is likely to obstruct actions aimed at enhancing the welfare of others who need one's help. However, the pursuit of achievement values may be compatible with the pursuit of power values: seeking personal success for oneself is likely to strengthen and to be strengthened by actions aimed at enhancing one's own social position and authority over others.

The conflicts and congruities among all the types of values yield an integrated structure of values. This structure can be summarized with two orthogonal dimensions. *Self- enhancement vs. self-transcendence:* On this dimension, the power and achievement value types oppose the universalism and benevolence value types. Both of the former emphasize pursuit of self-interests, whereas both of the latter involve concern for the welfare and interests of others. *Openness to change vs. conservatism:* On this dimension, the self-direction and stimulation value types oppose the security, conformity and tradition value types. Both of the former emphasize independent action, thought and feeling, and readiness for new experience, whereas all of the latter emphasize self-restriction, order and resistance to change. Hedonism shares elements of both openness and self-enhancement. This basic structure has been found in samples from a wide variety of cultures (Schwartz, 1992, 1994; Schwartz & Sagiv, 1995). It points to the broad underlying motivations that may constitute a universal principle that organizes value systems. People may differ substantially in the importance they attribute to values that comprise the ten value types, but their values are apparently organized by the same structure of motivational oppositions and compatibilities.

The version of the Schwartz Value Survey used for the present study is based on the so-called Portrait Version of the instrument (PVQ). It has 21 items modeled after the PVQ version used in the European Social Survey.[10] Gender versions were, however, not kept separate, but were collapsed into one version. Readers should note one more important change from the format used in the standard format of the PVQ. In the standard format, the instruction refers to an unnamed person with whom the respondent is to compare him or herself with regard to his/her value preferences.

10 http://www.europeansocialsurvey.org.

Table 1

Schwartz's Ten Motivational Types of Values (including sample items)

Power: Social status and prestige, control or dominance over people and resources	"It is important to him/her to be rich. He/she wants to have a lot of money and expensive things."
Achievement: Personal success through demonstrating competence according to social standards	"It's important to him/her to show his/her abilities. He/she wants people to admire what he/she does."
Hedonism: Pleasure or sensuous gratification for oneself	"Having a good time is important to him/her. He/she likes to "spoil" him/herself."
Stimulation: Excitement, novelty, and challenge in life	"He/she looks for adventures and likes to take risks. He/she wants to have an exciting life."
Self-Direction: Independent thought and action—choosing, creating, exploring	"Thinking up new ideas and being creative is important to him/her. He/she likes to do things in his/her own original way."
Universalism: Understanding, appreciation, tolerance, and protection for the welfare of all people and for nature	"It is important to him/her to listen to people who are different from him/her. Even when he/she disagrees with them, he/she still wants to understand them."
Benevolence: Preservation and enhancement of the welfare of people with whom one is in frequent personal contact	"It's very important to him/her to help the people around him/her. He/she wants to care for their wellbeing."
Tradition: Respect, commitment, and acceptance of the customs and ideas that traditional culture or religion provide	"It is important to him/her to be humble and modest. He/she tries not to draw attention to him or herself."
Conformity: Restraint of actions, inclinations, and impulses likely to upset or harm others and violate social expectations or norms	"He/she believes that people should do what they're told. He/she thinks people should follow rules at all times, even when no-one is watching."
Security: Safety, harmony, and stability of society, of relationships, and of self	"It is important to him/her that the government insure his/her safety against all threats. He/she wants the state to be strong so it can defend its citizens."

In the version used here, the person with whom a respondent is to make a comparison is labeled a "German person," a member of the "German people." This format was used for two reasons, one being the intention to force respondents to express value preferences with a clear focus on their own immigrant identity. The second reason was that by using this format, the mean rating of all items can at the same time be used as an overall acculturation index: The higher the score the more similar a respondent perceives him or herself to "the Germans."

4.4.3 Migration Attitude Questionnaire (MAQ)

The Migration Attitude Questionnaire was developed by the first author and was used to measure the general attitude concerning the experience of living in a new environment (see Table 2).

Table 2

Items of the Migration Attitude Questionnaire

#	Wording of Item
1	I have *been wasting away*
2	Compared to *before, economically* my situation has *improved*
3	I enjoy an *improved living standard*
4	The *cohesion* of my *family* is good
5	I experienced *police harassment*
6	I have felt *racial discrimination*
7	I sense *prejudice from Germans*
8	I have been confronted with *prejudice from fellow Africans*
9	I feel *socially backward*
10	*Living here is very stressful*
11	*I am happier than before*
12	*I am very sad*
13	*I want to go back home*
14	I have *no decent job*
15	*I am going through a lot of hassles*
16	*I want to live here forever*
17	*I am confused*
18	I *regretted* having *come here*
19	I admire *equal opportunities to job and health care*
20	I am *confronted with so many problems*

It is a 20-item self-report questionnaire; each question has five possible responses: 'not at all' (0), 'very little' (1), 'sometimes' (2), 'most of the time' (3), and 'all of the time' (4). The items were deliberately kept in a lingo common among English-speaking sub-Saharan Africans (in italics), but the table offers the items in a Standard English version. The exact formulation of the item can be taken from the Appendix of this volume.

The scale was pretested with 31 African migrants from the general population in Bremen to establish the consistency and validity of the Migration Attitude Questionnaire (MAQ). In the pretest the internal consistency of the scale (with appropriately reversed items) was high (overall alpha and standardized item alpha both were .86). This indicates that the MAQ is highly reliable for use among African migrants. The Migration Attitude Questionnaire was derived from reports on daily experiences of African migrants themselves, items were retained in the language used by migrants.

5. Socio-Demographic Characteristics of Respondents

The accounts of the socio-demographic characteristics of the study participants will be given for the overall sample, and—subsequently—for the general population and the prison subsample, separately.

5.1 Gender

In the overall sample, there were 26.6 % women and 73.4 % men. Tested by a binomial test the proportions differ significantly ($p < .001$). Among the participants from the general population, there were 34.5 % women and 65.5 % men. In the prison subsample, all but one were men (95.2 %). According to data from the German Federal Office of Statistics, the percentage of females among legal African residents of Germany in the year of study (2003) was 36.9 %.[11] In the present sample from the general population the percentage was just slightly lower, but considering the fact that considerable numbers of illegal immigrants were also included, who presumably are in the vast majority males, suggests that the gender proportions of the general population subsample are representative for Africans in Germany. The fact that in the prison subsample there are only 4.8 % women also comes very close to being representative for the actual gender distribution of prison inmates. In 2006, 5.3 % of all German prison inmates were women (Cornel, 2007). Given that the African population has fewer women to begin with, 4.8 % perfectly matches the expected figure.

5.2 Age

The mean age of the full sample is 31.65 with a standard deviation of 7.31. In the general population subsample the age is 31.60 with a standard devia-

[11] https://www-ec.destatis.de/csp/shop/sfg/bpm.html.cms.cBroker.cls?cmspath=struktur, vollanzeige.csp&ID= 1024112

tion of 7.09; in the inmate subsample the average age is 31.79 with a standard deviation of 8.16. The average age of the two subsamples does not differ significantly ($p > .25$). Figure 2 documents the age distribution of the study participants.

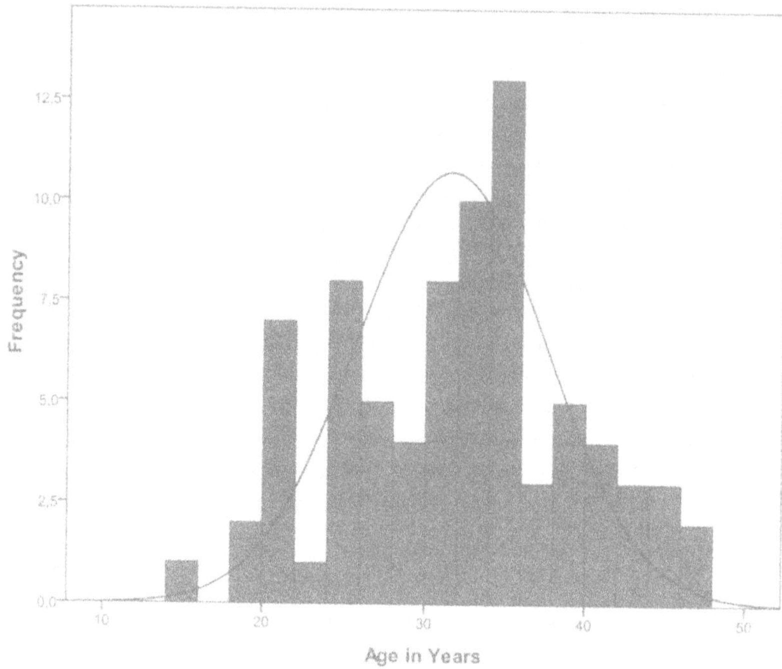

Figure 2: *Age Distribution of the Full Sample*

In 2008 the average age of legal African residents of Germany is reported to be 34.1, likely to have increased slightly from the time the survey was conducted[12]. Once again it can be assumed that the average age of the current sample is representative for Africans living in Germany, regardless of their legal status, because it seems plausible to assume that illegal immigrants are

12 https://www-ec.destatis.de/csp/shop/sfg/bpm.html.cms.cBroker.cls?cmspath=struktur,vollanzeige.csp&ID= 1015274

of a somewhat younger age, so that the average age of 31.7 reflects the typical age of African immigrants to Germany very well.

5.3 Marital Status

In the overall sample 38.1 % were single, 34.6 % were either separated or divorced, and 27.4 % were married. Percentages differed in a marginally significant way (p = .097) between the two subsamples—in a somewhat surprising manner: In the general population sample 35.5 % were single, 42.0 % were separated or divorced, and only 22.6 % were married, whereas in the inmate subsample 45.5 % were single, only 13.6 % were separated or divorced, and 40.9 % were married.

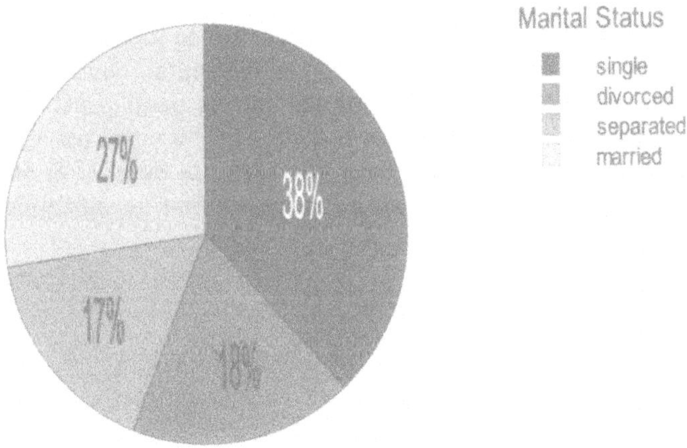

Figure 3: *Marital Status (Percentages, rounded)*

An assessment as to whether these percentages are representative for Africans residing in Germany is difficult. Data for the end of 2008 suggest that 46.0 % of African legal residents of Germany were single, 40.0 % were married, 6.7 % were divorced, 1.0 % were widowed and 6.3 % were of unknown marital status. First of all, the situation may have changed slightly between the year of the survey and 2008, but no sufficiently exact data could be obtained for 2003. Secondly, no comparative data is available for illegal immigrants, and thirdly it is difficult to determine, how people who in our survey indicated that they were separated would formally have been categorized in the official statistic. It does seem likely, however, that our sample of legal and illegal African residents of Germany has more divorcees and separated individuals than is the case in a sample of legal residents only. This results of analyses of the socio-demographic data makes it necessary—and interesting—to take a special look at differences in acculturative stress, value preferences, and mental health according to marital status. Figure 3 documents the distribution of marital status in the overall sample.

5.4 Educational and Professional Attainment

Current levels of educational attainment are as follows in the grand sample: Some 9.2 % have only primary or no education, down from 10.5 % upon arrival to Germany. Exactly one half of the participants have a secondary education (or equivalent), down from 56.6 % upon arrival. At least some post-secondary education have 14.5 %, up from 11.8 % upon arrival, whereas 26.3 % have completed at least a first university degree) up from 21.1 %.

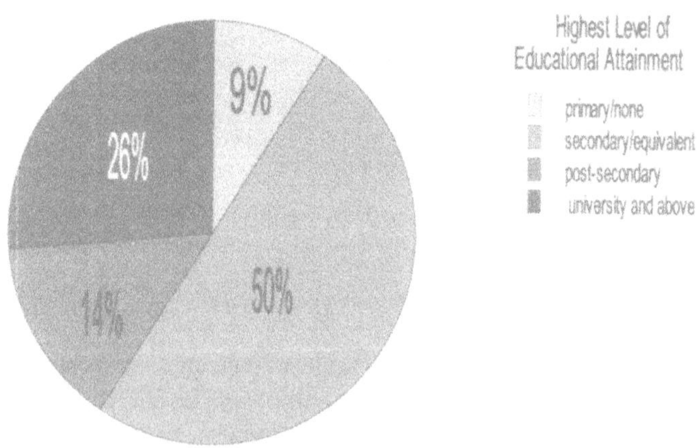

Figure 4: *Levels of Educational Attainment (Percentages, rounded)*

Differences in educational attainment between the general population sample and the inmate sample were significant; Wilcoxon's W was significant (p=.048): educational attainment was lower in the inmate subsample. Figure 4 documents the distribution of educational attainment levels in the grand sample.

As documented in Figure 5, 12.9 % of all participants were students at the time of surveying, 18.8 % had skilled professional occupations, a relative majority of 37.6 % held skilled non-professional jobs, 11.8 % were employed in unskilled jobs, whereas 18.8 % of the respondents were unemployed. Also here the sample seems to be fairly representative for the population of African migrants residing in Germany. Grundig and Pohl (2006) report that in 2003 the percentage of unemployed among migrants in Germany is about twice as high as among German nationals, the latter being around 9 %, the prior around 17 %. More detailed data for African migrants to Germany could not be obtained, so that one has to take the overall data for migrants as a point of reference. Between participants from the general population distributions of professional attainment different highly significantly (p<.001): Among the unemployed prison inmates are much more frequent than among general population participants. Relative proportions and absolute frequencies of the different occupations in the two subsamples are documented in Figure 5.

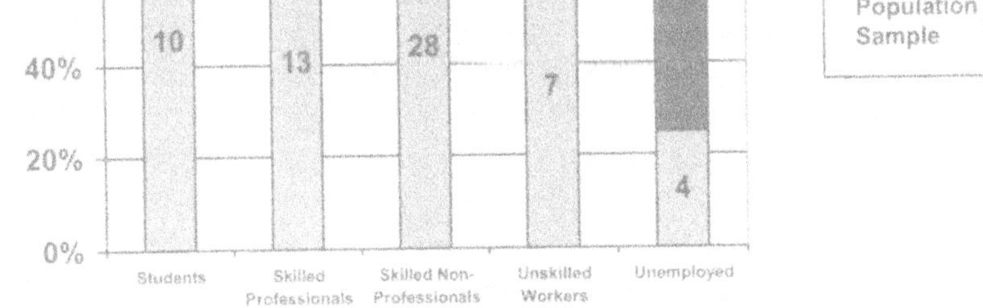

Figure 5: *Relative and Absolute Frequencies of Occupations of Respondents*

5.5 Country of Upbringing, Migration Motivation, and Duration of Stay in Germany

The participants were also asked to indicate from where they migrated to Germany. Due to eased accessibility for the first author, a Nigerian national, a majority of respondents came from Nigeria (56.5 %). More than a single respondent was interviewed from Ghana (9.4 %), Senegal (4.7 %), Kenya, Congo (Kinshasa), and Togo (2.4 %, each). Some 13 % came from other African countries, while more than 9 % of the respondents refused to indicate their country of upbringing. If a study includes illegal immigrants from Africa, obtaining nationalities seems to be a 'tricky' issue. Considerable numbers of respondent are unwilling to disclose their country of upbringing even in an anonymous survey.

As for reasons to migrate to Germany, 40.5 % indicated economic problems at home as the main reason, 20.3 % came for reasons of political problems at home, 19.0 % came to study in Germany, 11.4 % sought work (without indicating economic problems at home), and 8.9 % came for family reasons (one or the other type of family reunion as the main reason). Relative proportions are documented in Figure 6.

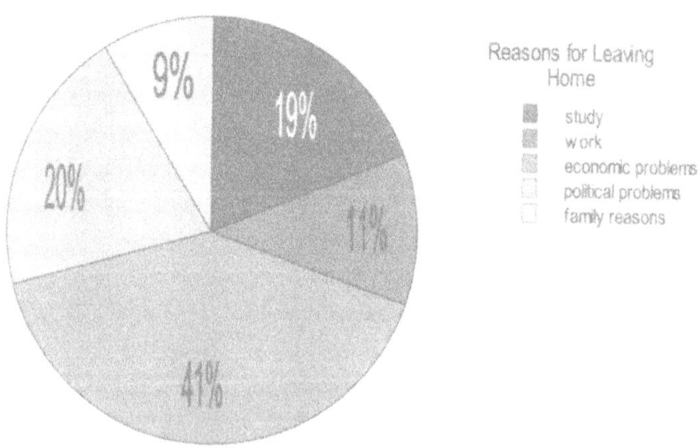

Figure 6: *Migration Motives (Percentages, rounded)*

As for the number of years participants have stayed in Germany, answers had a considerable range, varying between half a year and 20 years. The average duration of stay in Germany was 7.46 years with a standard deviation of 4.51 years. Figure 7 documents details. The duration of stay in Germany did not differ between the general population subsample and the prison inmate subsample. However, there are significant differences in the duration of stay in Germany ($p = .001$) according to level of educational attainment: Immigrants with only primary or no education have stayed in Germany for a shorter time. Also are there significant differences in duration of stay between the different occupational groups ($p = .003$), with students and unskilled workers having stayed for a shorter period of time. There are marginally significant differences ($p = .065$) according to migration motivation in duration of stay, migrants who have come to study having stayed for the shortest, migrants who have come because of economic problems at home having stayed for the longest period of time.

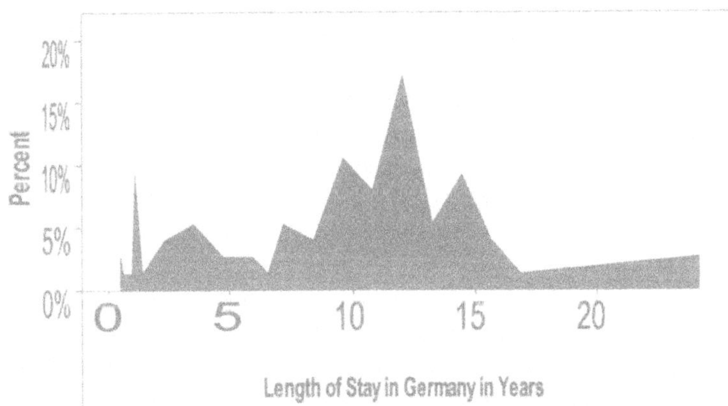

Figure 7: *Duration of Stay in Germany*

6. Self-Reported Migration Experience in Germany

Chapter 6 first reports descriptive evidence obtained with the Migration Attitude Questionnaire (MAQ). In order to make use of a maximum amount of data, missing values were imputed using an Expected Maximum algorithm, as offered by SPSS. Imputed values were in a second step truncated to scores between 0 and 4 (as offered in the rating format for MAQ questions).

At the end of the chapter, the overall evaluation of the stay in Germany, as provided in the open questions of Section A of the questionnaire booklet, will also be reported and related to results obtained with the MAQ.

Table 3 gives means and standard deviations for the 20 MAQ items in the order of descending means, i.e., from the item that drew highest approval to the onc that drew least approval. The table shows that the most pressing problem of African immigrants to Germany is that they see themselves as having no decent job. Somewhat surprisingly, no gender differences and no differences between the general population subsample and the prison inmate subsample were found ($p > .25$).

For further analyses an index variable was formed that is assumed to measure the overall degree of acculturative stress cxpcricnccd by the surveyed immigrants. The development of this index variable was based on an exploratory factor analysis—details omitted here. All those items that had its highest loadings on the strong first factor of the scale (*eigenvalue* 9.215) were averaged for the calculation of the index variable (after appropriate recoding if pertinent). Items 1, 5, 6, 7, 9, 10, 12, 13, 14, 15, 17, 18, 19 (reversed), and 20 were used to form the index variable (for details readers should refer to Table 2 and 3). The index variable had a mean of 2.39 with a standard deviation of 1.14. Consistency of the acculturative stress variable was very high; Cronbach's alpha was .95.

Acculturative stress can reasonably be assumed to decrease in the course of a longer stay. It seems logical to assume that something like a culture shock should be strongest in the beginning of a migrant's stay in a new culture. For African immigrants to Germany, however, the opposite is true: The longer they stay in Germany, the more acculturative stress they express. By correcting for a respondent's age, that is, correcting for the possibility that the older someone gets, the more stressed he or she feels, it can be shown that it is indeed the duration of stay that lets the experience of stress become stronger and not increasing age: A multiple regression analysis with both duration of stay and age in years as predictors of the degree of acculturative stress, emphasizes that it is the duration of stay ($ß = .33$, $p = .014$) and not the respondent's age ($ß = .04$, $p = .779$) that is significantly positively related to acculturative stress. It seems plausible to assume that the longer Africans stay in Germany, the more stressed they feel.

Table 3

Means of the Migration Attitude Questionnaire

Items (#)	Mean	Standard Deviation
No decent job (14)	2.71	1.421
Lots of hassles (15)	2.65	1.396
Economically improved (2)	2.65	1.381
Very stressful life (10)	2.65	1.363
Racial discrimination (6)	2.65	1.395
Many problems (20)	2.64	1.300
Improved living standard (3)	2.60	1.063
Happier than before (11)	2.58	1.380
Prejudice from Germans (7)	2.38	1.385
Wasting away (1)	2.35	1.685
Family cohesion (4)	2.32	1.274
Very sad (12)	2.23	1.515
Confused (17)	2.15	1.527
Police harassment (5)	2.11	1.637
Go back home (13)	2.05	1.291
Regretted having come (18)	2.03	1.566
Socially backward (9)	1.97	1.581
Prejudice from Africans (8)	1.36	1.135
Live here forever (16)	1.34	1.259
Equal opportunities (19)	1.16	1.332

In subsequent analyses we corrected for differences in both age and duration of stay, in order to obtain 'pure' results for the further effects that we tested, not results that might have their origin in difference in age and duration of stay.

As for marital status, distinct differences were found for the different status groups ($p < .01$). It clearly emerged that divorced and separated respondents reported considerably higher acculturative stress than respondents who were either single or married. Figure 8 documents details.

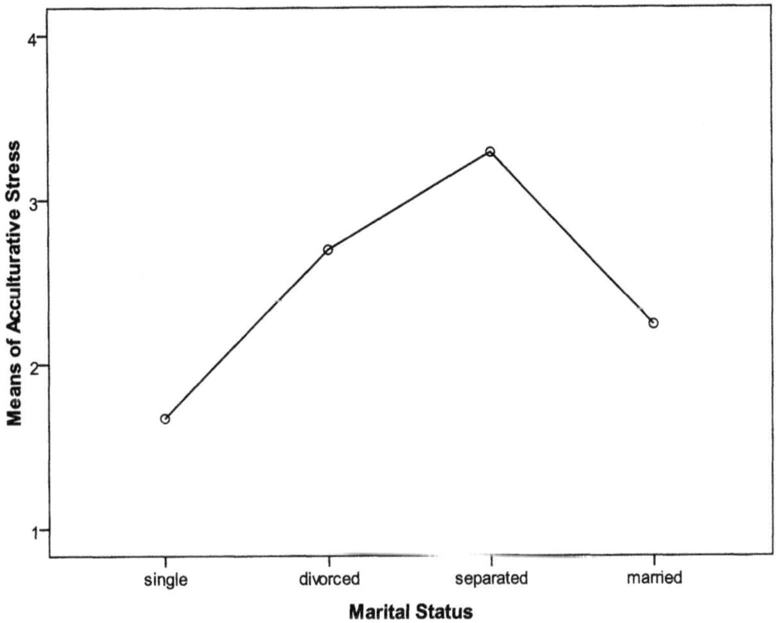

Figure 8: *Acculturative Stress as a Function of Marital Status*

The relationship between marital status and acculturative stress as documented in Figure 8, does, however, need amendment. If one checks whether the finding holds for both males and females, it emerges that divorced women, but separated men report the highest levels of acculturative stress. Divorced men, on the contrary, report lowest levels of stress among all marital status groups ($p <. 001$). Figure 9 reports details.

Divorced men report a level of acculturative stress that makes them very similar to their single fellow migrants, whereas divorced women can probably be said to face an existential crisis.

A further possible source of variation in acculturative stress is one's level of educational attainment. It is difficult to predict whether people with higher levels of education will express more acculturative stress or people with lower levels. Life will typically tend to be 'harder' for people with low levels of educational attainment. Acculturative stress, however, has a strong perceptual component, suggesting that also people with higher levels of education may after all experience more stress, because they are, on the one hand, more differentiated in their perception and, on the other hand, may be more easily disappointed about their factual accomplishments given their higher levels of education.

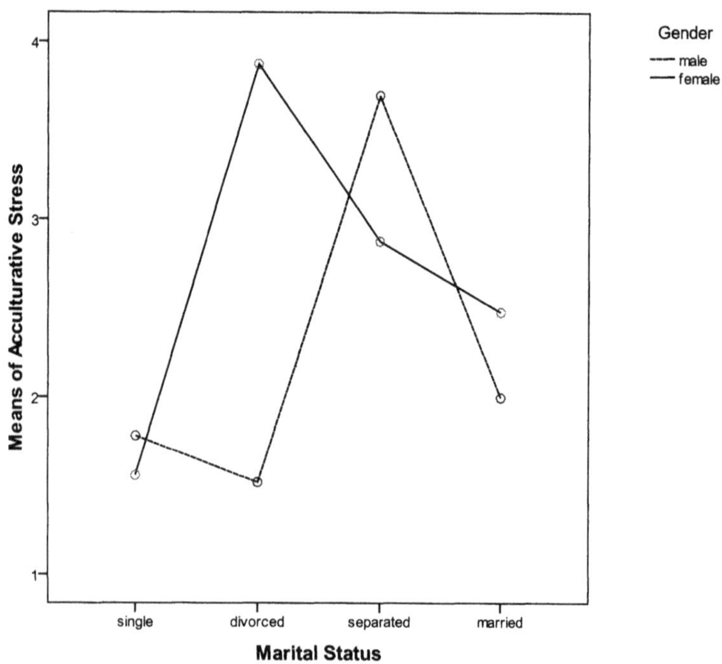

Figure 9: *Acculturative Stress as a Function of Marital Status* (♀/♂)

Figure 10 documents that men do not differ substantially according to their levels of educational attainment. Women with a secondary or equivalent level of education suffer most, while women with only primary or no education as well as women with a university degree report least acculturative stress.

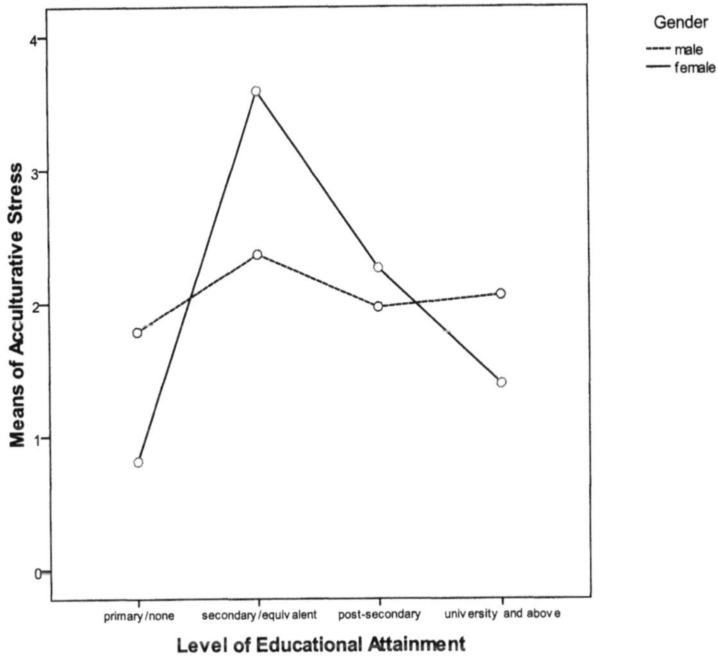

Figure 10: *Acculturative Stress as a Function of Educational Attainment* (♀/♂)

When looking at differences in acculturative stress according to present occupations, the ambiguous meaning of self-reported acculturative stress once again becomes obvious: Least stress is—not surprisingly—reported by students, but acculturative stress reported by unemployed African immigrants is almost identically low. Highest acculturative stress is reported by skilled non-professionals ($p = .003$), probably the group that has the most genuine contact with locals. Figure 11 documents pertinent details.

Finally, differences in the migration motivation of African immigrants may have an impact on acculturative stress, and they indeed do ($p < .001$). Figure 12 shows that having come to study, for political, or for family reasons goes along with relatively little acculturative stress, whereas having come for work or because of economic problems at home goes along with high acculturative stress.

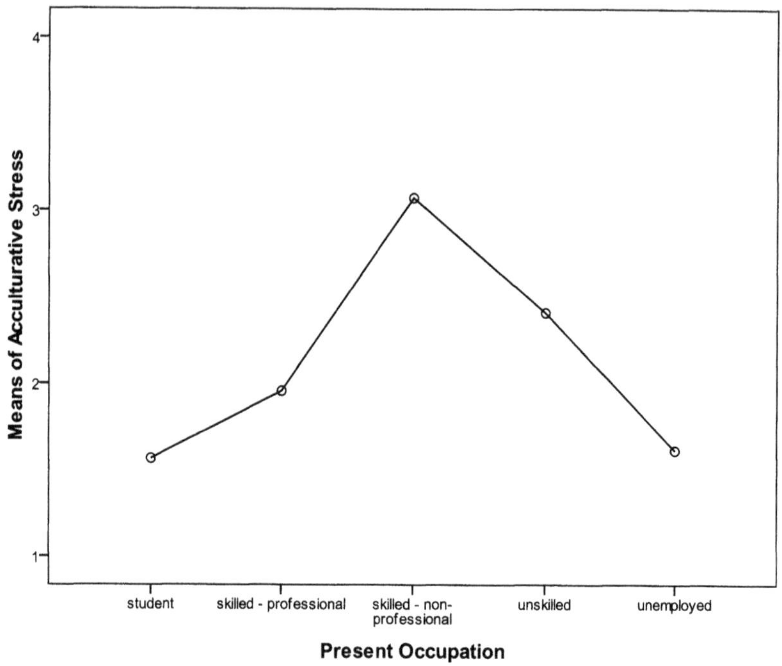

Figure 11: *Acculturative Stress as a Function of Present Occupation*

In a concluding step, a hierarchic regression analysis was performed. In it all variables included in the prior analyses of predictors of acculturative stress were entered into the regression equation in blocks. To accommodate for the relatively small sample size of the study, within blocks only variables that were at least marginally significantly related to the dependent variable 'acculturative stress' ($p < .10$) were included, using the STEPWISE procedure. The analyses showed that 52.2 % (adjusted R^2) of the variance in acculturative stress is explained by the variables in the final equation. In substantive terms this means that more than one half of the acculturative stress of African migrants is explained by the variables tested in the analysis, most significantly as to whether migrants were separated ($ß = .35$, $p = .001$), came for reasons of economic problems at home ($ß = .34$, $p = .004$), were divorced ($ß = .29$, $p = .007$), or came to seek work ($ß = .15$, $p = .093$).

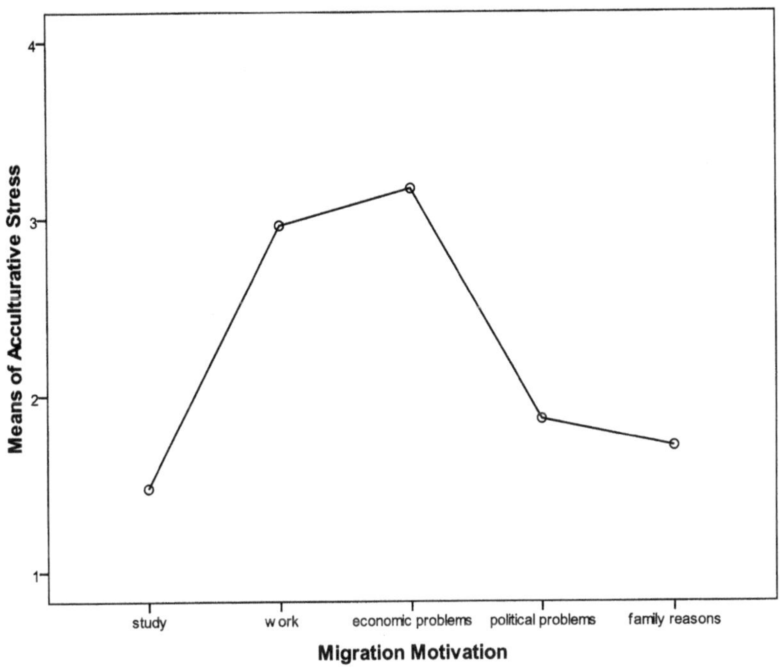

Figure 12: *Acculturative Stress as a Function of Migration Motivation*

When asked for an overall evaluation of their experience in Germany, 48.5 % of all responses could be coded as 'negative,' 20 % as 'neutral,' and 31.5 % as 'positive.' When asked of what nature problems were that they had incurred in Germany, about one quarter of the respondents did not report any problems or explicitly indicated that they had never had any. On the other hand, a good third of the respondents reported problems with racial discrimination. The remaining some 40 % of the respondents reported various other problems. When asked whether they had had problems with the law in Germany, 40 % of all respondents indicated that they had had such problems, with 43.8 % of them reporting criminal offenses as the reason for the problems. These data—from open questions—validate findings obtained with the acculturative stress measure: Acculturative stress and the overall assessment of the 'German experience' correlated significantly with each other. Kendall's τ_b rank correlation was .37 ($p < .001$). The correlation of acculturative stress and self-reported problems with racial discrimination was of a comparable size ($\tau_b = .32$, $p < .001$).

In a nutshell results of the analyses presented in Chapter 6 can be summarized as showing that being separated from one's spouse and having come as an economic refugee are the most prominent sources of acculturative stress of African migrants in Germany. Having no decent job, being overburdened with hassles and problems, and racial discrimination by Germans are the most prominent sources of stress.

7. Mental Health Status

Chapter 7 offers descriptive evidence on the mental health status of the overall sample by reporting MMPI-2 scores for the following subscales: Anxiety, Depression, Health Concerns, Bizarre Mentation, Anger, Social Discomfort, Family Problems, Work Interference, Low Self-Esteem, and Negative Treatment Indicators. As for scoring, two options were discussed by the authors. One was the classical option where all yes-answers were scored '1' and were then added up, with both no-answers and missing answers counted as '0.' The other option was to also score yes-answers as '1' and no-answers as '0,' but then only add up all valid responses, divide by the number of valid responses and multiply by the number of items in the scale. In substantive terms the latter procedure counts missing answers as yes-answers to the proportions of yes-answers given by a respondent to non-missing items of a scale. The subsequent report will document classical scores. In no instance did the alternative scores yield substantively different results.

Table 4 documents the average scale scores for the 10 MMPI scales used in the present study (in the order of descending means).

Table 4
Scales Scores for MMPI Scales Used in the Present Study

MMPI Scale	Mean	Standard Deviation
Depression	13.12	8.33
Health Problems	11.60	4.59
Work Interference	10.07	6.25
Anxiety	9.93	4.87
Bizarre Mentation	9.16	6.29
Low Self-Esteem	9.15	6.62
Family Problems	9.07	5.64
Social Discomfort	7.86	3.76
Negative Treatment Indicators	5.73	4.14
Anger	4.96	3.14

The table shows that the most relevant mental health predicaments pertain to depression, (somatic and psychosomatic) health problems, and problems that interfere with the migrant's ability to work properly.

We first checked whether mental health scores differed between men and women, and between the general population subsample and the prison inmate subsample. In order to test for these differences, we performed a multivariate two-way analysis of variance (MANOVA) with subsequent univariate tests for the 10 subscales. Analyses show that there is a significant multivariate gender effect ($p = .020$), a significant 'inmate' effect ($p = .002$), and a marginally significant gender-by-'inmate' interaction effect (p =. 080). The latter should, however, not be taken all that serious, because there was only one incarcerated woman in the sample. When looking at the single scales, we found only few significant effects. Women had slightly higher scores on the anger and the negative treatment indicators subscales ($p = .073$/$p = .087$). On all other scales men and women did not differ significantly. As for inmate vs. non-inmates, they differed on the low self-esteem scale, inmates surprisingly reporting significantly lower scores ($p = .026$), suggesting that their self-reported self-esteem is indeed higher.

As we did for acculturative stress, we again checked for the relationship between age, duration of stay in Germany, and our mental health indicators by performing multiple regression analyses with age and duration of stay as predictors and the ten mental health scales (separately) as dependent variables. Table 5 documents standardized regression coefficients for both predictors for the ten mental health scales. It shows that for eight out of ten scales, scores were significantly higher the longer the migrants had stayed in Germany, regardless of their age. In no single case did chronological age have a significant genuine impact on the mental scores. In spite of the fact that our study certainly does not allow causal interpretations, this is indication, for a second time, that staying in Germany longer adds to poor mental health scores of African migrants, or put in an overly plain language, that Germany makes them sick.

In further analytic steps we tested, also for mental health, whether scores differed by marital status, educational attainment, present occupation, and migration motivation. In order to test for these effects we performed multivariate analyses of covariance (MANCOVA) separately for the four different independent variables, and age and duration of stay in Germany as covariates, the 10 MMPI scales being the multivariate dependent variables. Subsequently univariate tests were performed for the separate scales in cases where the multivariate effects proved significant.

Table 5

MMPI Scales Scores as Predicted by Age and Duration of Stay in Germany

MMPI Scale	Age in Years *ß*	Duration of Stay in Germany *ß*
Depression	-.19	.39**
Health Problems	-.04	.29*
Work Interference	-.10	.32*
Anxiety	-.08	.36**
Bizarre Mentation	-.06	.39**
Low Self-Esteem	-.03	.24
Family Problems	-.04	.39**
Social Discomfort	-.02	.19
Negative Treatment Indicators	-.08	.33*
Anger	-.15	.27*

For all ten scales mental health scores differed significantly ($p \leq .001$) between the four categories of marital status. The rank order of scores always was the same: Separated respondents had highest scores, followed by divorced, married, and single respondents. The strongest effect of marital status was found for the depression scale. Figure 13 documents details.

For 'educational attainment' effects were substantially smaller ($p = .050$), but also here scores for all 10 mental health scales differed at least marginally significantly. For all scales, migrants who have completed secondary schooling or equivalent exhibited highest scores when compared to migrants with only primary or no education, with at least some post-secondary education, or holding a university degree. Means of the other educational attainment groups differed from scale to scale in their rank order. The strongest effect emerged again for the depression scale. Figure 14 documents details.

For 'present occupation' effects were multivariately quite strong ($p = .002$), but univariately significant effects were found 'only' for eight out of ten scales. No significant occupation differences were found for Health Problems and for Social Discomfort. The strongest effect was this time found for Low Self-Esteem. Figure 15 documents details.

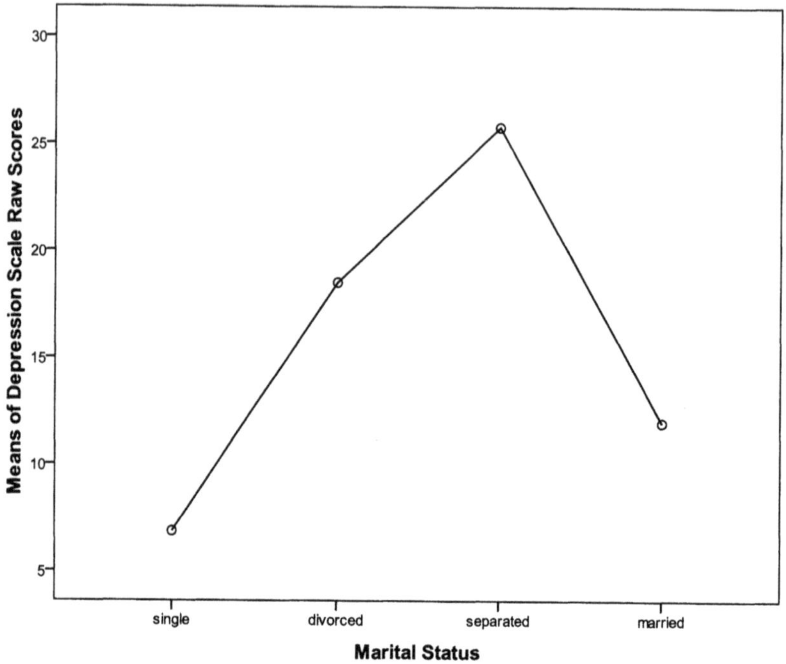

Figure 13: *Depression Scores as a Function of Marital Status*

It is interesting to note that Low Self-Esteem is *not* reported most pronouncedly by unemployed migrants. They on the contrary had lowest scores on this scale, meaning that they reported a fairly high self-esteem. We will discuss this finding in the concluding chapter of this volume.

Furthermore, mental health scores also differed strongly multivariately as a function of migration motivation ($p < .001$). Univariately, significant motivation differences ($p < .05$) were found for all ten scales. The strongest effect again emerged for the Low Self-Esteem scale. Migrants who came for reasons of economic problems at home or just to seek work in Germany exhibited highest scores on this scale, thereby reporting strong self-esteem deficits. Details are given in Figure 16.

In a concluding analytic step we once again set out to determine which predictors were the relatively strongest among the independent variables scrutinized above. We performed another hierarchic regression analysis. In it all variables included in the prior analyses of predictors of mental health were entered into the regression equation in blocks. To accommodate for the relatively small sample size of the study, within blocks once again only variables that were at least marginally significantly related to the mental health scale score under scrutiny in an analysis (p <. 10) were included, using the STEPWISE procedure. Table 6 gives an overview of significant predictors of the ten MMPI scale raw scores.

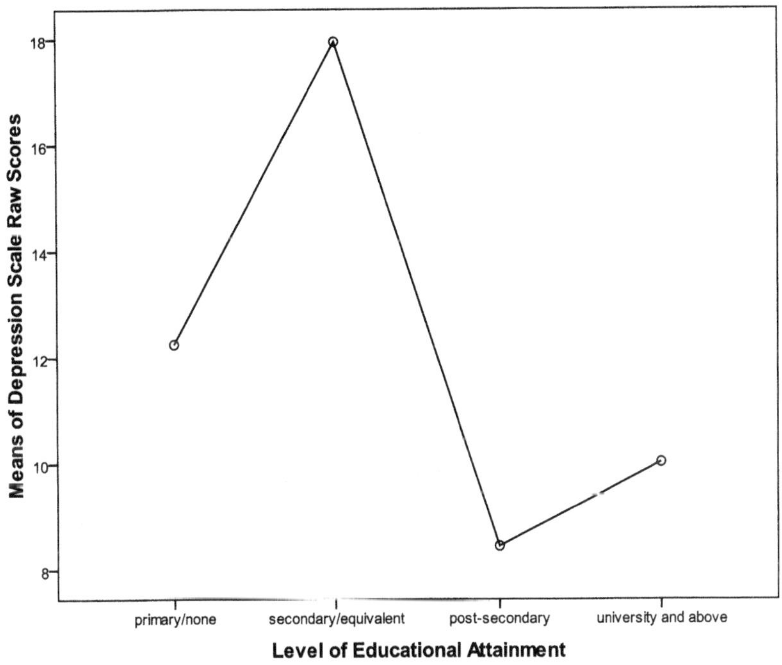

Figure 14: *Depression Scores as a Function of Educational Attainment*

Table 6 clearly indicates that for an African Migrant, living in Germany as a separated or divorced individual has the relatively strongest risk potential for the migrant's mental health. Also, having come with secondary education only poses a risk. Having come for family reasons, i.e., having migrated for reasons of some sort of family reunion, serves as a protection factor.

In summary it can be said that African migrants residing in Germany do not enjoy a very good mental health status, to say the least. Although no comprehensive norm tables are available for Africans, and particularly not for

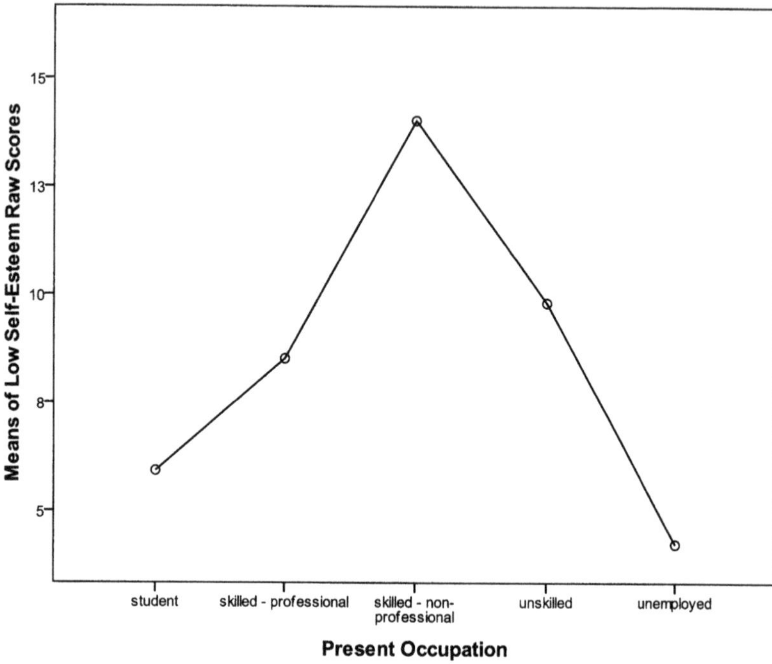

Figure 15: *Low Self-Esteem Scores as a Function of Present Occupation*

Africans in the Diaspora, an educated guess suggests that a quarter of the surveyed respondents has clinically relevant mental health problems: Their T-values (the standard values calculated from the MMPI raw scores) are above 70 on one or more of the MMPI scales included in the present study. After a brief report on value preferences of African migrants, the remainder of the volume will focus on the question whether this to be seen as a consequence of the acculturative life experience in Germany or as corollary of a selection process that seduces individuals into migration who are from the very beginning of a poorer mental health status. Of course, the present study is not designed in a way to offer decisive evidence on this principled question, but in case "socialization," that is, the experience in Germany, had a stronger impact, acculturative stress should be a stronger direct predictor of mental health than predictors like migration motivation or education attainment. We will be addressing this question is Chapter 9.

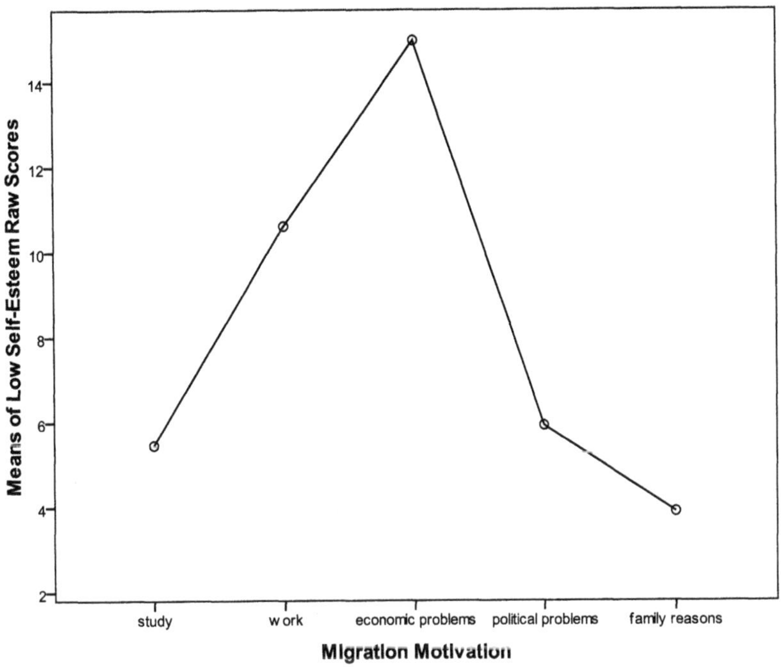

Figure 16: *Low Self-Esteem Scores as a Function of Migration Motivation*

Table 6

Predictors of Mental Health

MMPI Scale	Marital Status: 'separated'	Marital Status: 'divorced'	Marital Status: 'married'	Educational Attainment: 'secondary'	Migration Motivation: 'family reasons'	Migration Motivation: 'economic problems'	Migration Motivation: 'work'	Female Gender	Inmate
DEP	.51***			.28**	-.22*			.26**	
HEA	.40***	.40***							
WRK	.53***	.21*	.24*	.21*				.32***	-.24**
ANX	.34***			.37***	-.25**				
BIZ	.48***	.30**			-.19*				
LSE	.41***	.31***		.25**		.29*	.17*		
FAM	.46***	.24*							
SOD				.42***					-.32*
TRY	.43***			.26**	-.28**			.26*	
ANG	.38***								

8. Value Preferences

Value preferences of respondents were obtained by a modified PVQ version of the Schwartz Value Survey (see Chapter 4). Chapter 8 offers descriptive evidence on preferences expressed by the survey African migrants residing in Germany.

Table 7 documents raw mean scores for the ten value scales in the order they are arranged in Schwartz's value theory.

Table 7
Means of the Ten Schwartz Value Types

Value Type	Mean	Standard Deviation	Rank
Universalism	4.75	1.23	2
Benevolence	4.30	1.20	7
Tradition	4.21	1.19	8
Conformity	4.55	1.17	3
Security	4.79	1.25	1
Power	4.35	1.29	6
Achievement	4.37	1.15	5
Hedonism	3.81	1.18	9
Stimulation	3.74	1.33	10
Self-Direction	4.42	1.13	4

Means of the present version of the PVQ should not at face value be compared with means obtained with the original version of the PVQ in other samples. It is, however, obvious that respondents emphasized security and conformity values much more than would be common in a German sample (Cohrs, Moschner, Maes, & Kielmann, 2005).

The first analytic step once again pertained to gender and to the comparison of inmates and respondents from the general population. Also here, a multivariate analysis of variance was performed with the independent variables gender and 'inmate,' and the ten value types as dependent variables. Following advice by Schwartz (1992), the mean rating per person across all value items is used as a covariate in this analysis to correct for—idiosyncratic—scale use. It emerged that there is no significant difference in the value preferences of the general population and the inmate subsample ($p > .25$), whereas a gender ($p = .022$) and a gender-by-inmate interaction ($p = .022$) were found. The latter should, however, once again not be taken very serious due to the fact that there was only one woman amongst the surveyed inmates. Gender differences were significant for universalism ($p = .013$, men higher) and hedonism values ($p = .019$, women higher), and marginally significant for power ($p = .093$, women higher), achievement ($p = .060$; men higher), and stimulation values ($p = .066$, women higher).

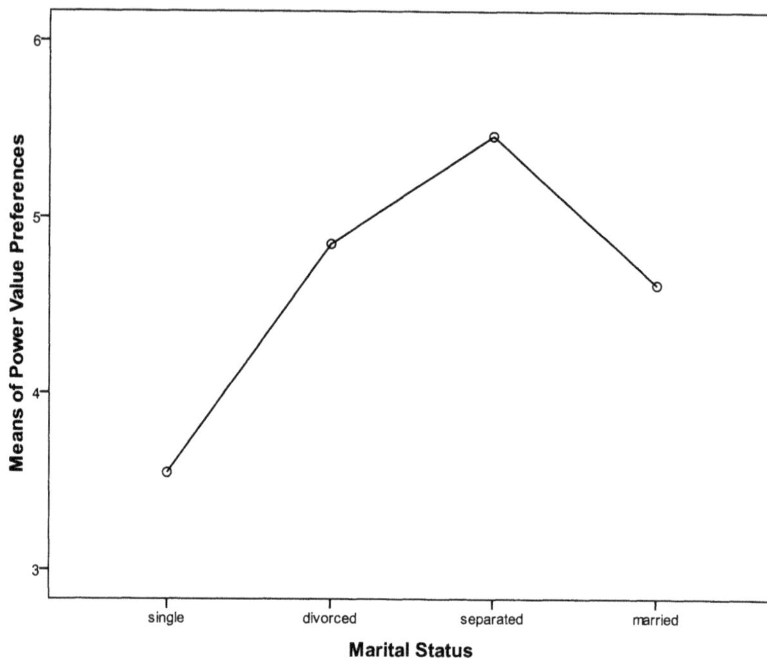

Figure 17: *Power Value Preferences as a Function of Marital Status*

Duration of stay in Germany and age were next checked for a relationship with value preferences in the same manner as described just above. It showed that hardly any relationship exists. Conformity is significantly related to the respondent's age ($ß = .29$, $p = .004$), conformity being preferred more among older respondents. Preferences for benevolence values are slightly higher among the young ($ß = -.17$, $p = .065$), and stimulation values are preferred by respondents who have stayed in Germany longer ($ß = .17$, $p = .086$).

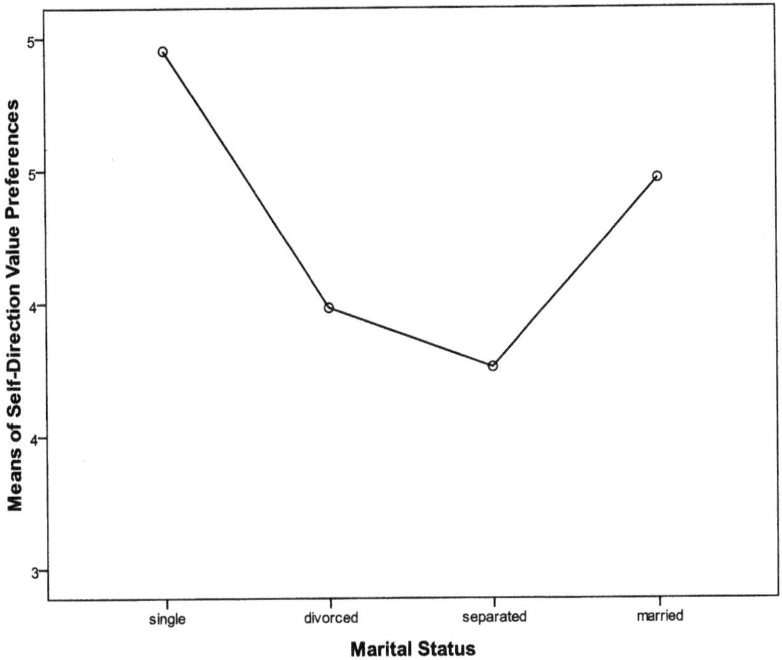

Figure 18: *Self-Direction Value Preferences as a Function of Marital Status*

As for marital status, a multivariate main effect was found (p = .027), but only for two value types univariate differences could be corroborated, power values (p <.001) and self-direction values (p = .007). Details for both values are documented in Figure 17 and 18. The figures show that preferences for both value types emerge as mirroring each other: Power values are particularly high among separated and divorced respondents, while self-determination values are particularly high among single and married respondents.

No significant effect of educational attainment level on value preferences was found (p > .25).

Value preferences did, however, differ between occupational groups (p = .004). At least marginally significant univariate differences (p < .10) between occupational groups were found for benevolence, tradition, achievement, and self-direction values. Differences for self-direction values were most pronounced; they are documented in Figure 19. Somewhat surprisingly, self-direction value preferences are least preferred in the two groups with skilled (professional or non-professional) occupations.

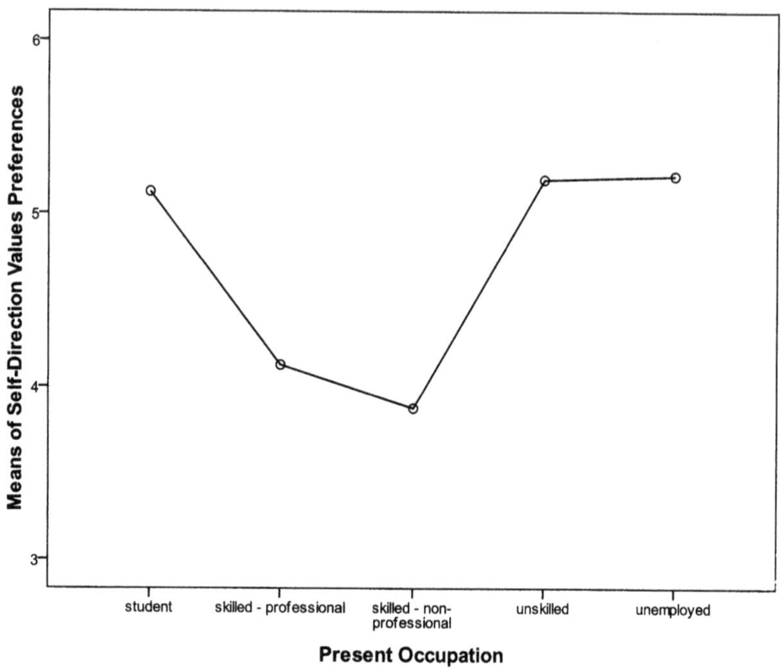

Figure 19: *Self-Direction Value Preferences as a Function of Present Occupation*

Value preferences also differed between according to migration motivation ($p = .001$). Al least marginally significant univariate differences ($p < .10$) between groups with different migration motivations were found for universalism, power, and self-direction values.

In this case (see Figure 20) differences in benevolence values emerged as most pronounced. Among migrants who left home to study in Germany, for political, or for family reasons, benevolence value preferences were considerably higher than in the group of migrants who came for reasons of economic problems at home or to seek work.

The final analytic step in reference to value preferences once again is that of a hierarchic regression analysis, performed analogously to the analyses reported for the mental health scales, only that this time, mean ratings across all value types were also partialled for. We refrain from documenting coefficients in detail here. When looking only at strong predictors (ß > .30) it emerges that only power and self-direction value preferences have clear predictive patterns: Power values are highest among all non-single marital status groups and among women, and particularly low among prison inmates. Self-direction values are particularly low among migrants who have a skilled job (professionals and non-professionals).

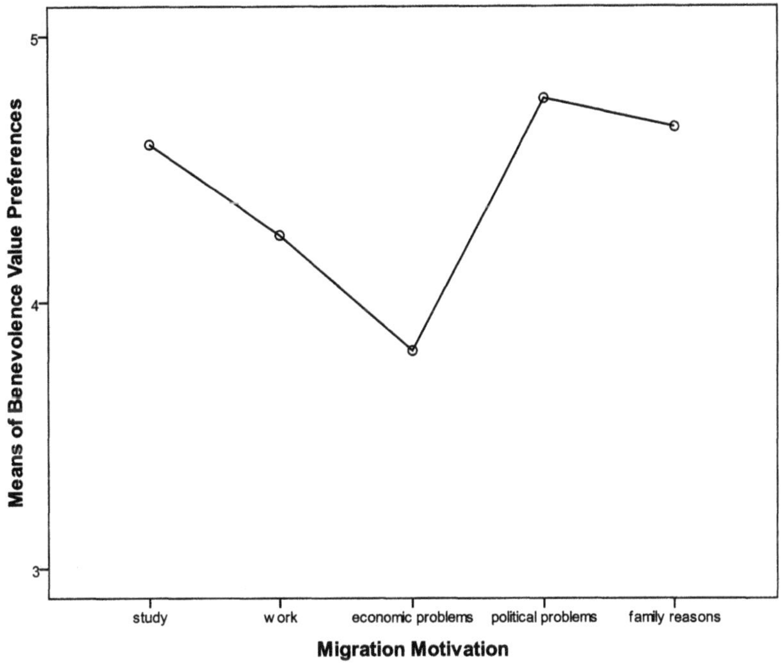

Figure 20: *Benevolence Value Preferences as a Function of Migration Motivation*

9. Acculturative Stress, Perceived Racism, and Mental Health

Chapter 9 inspects the relationship between acculturative stress and mental health. In order to obtain a comprehensive impression, scales scores of the MMPI were collapsed into one overall mental health indicator. The overall indicator was highly consistent: Cronbach's alpha emerged as .96 for the ten scale scores as 'meta'-items of a global mental health indicator.

To document the interrelation between sociodemographics, acculturative stress, racism, and overall mental health, a structural equation model (SEM) with the so-called *exogenous variables* 'age,' 'duration of stay in Germany,' 'gender,' 'separatedness' (as the respondent's marital status), 'secondary schooling' (as the level of educational attainment), and 'economic problems at home' (as the main migration motive), acculturative stress and perceived German racism as *mediator variables*, and overall poor mental health as the *criterion*.

The result of the pertinent analysis is depicted in Figure 21.

Correlations of exogenous variables and error terms of the mediator variables and the criterion are omitted from the figure. Table 8 offers standardized total, direct, and indirect effects for the prediction of poor overall mental health. All paths are significant ($p < .05$).

SEM analyses, as documented in Figure 21 and Table 8, offer the following evidence. Acculturative stress is a strong predictor of a migrant's mental health. Almost 50 percent of the variance in mental health scores are determined by the degree of self-reported acculturative stress. Perceived racism is a significant, but much weaker predictor of poor mental health. Additionally it should be emphasized that perceived racism does not itself add to the acculturative stress reported by migrants! Living a life separated from one's spouse, be it legally or through migration, and having had economic problems at home as the primary migration motive have a strong indirect negative impact on migrants' mental health as both add considerably to perceived acculturative stress. Having migrated for reasons of economic problems at home also increases the perception of racism in Germany. Obviously those migrants who are self-labeled economic refugees are confronted most with German racism. Women suffer more from acculturative stress, but no genuine direct gender effect on mental health could be corroborated. As already highlighted earlier, and against logical expectations, staying longer in Germany adds to the experience of acculturative stress. Two direct effects of a sociodemographics variable on mental health were found, one for secondary schooling as the level of education attainment, the other for chronological age. One might interpret the prior finding as indication for a certain selection effect in migration moves, namely that those migrants who have not obtained a higher amount of schooling are already in a poorer mental state when they migrate as compared to their better educated (or for that matter even yet less educated) fellow migrants. The finding for age is difficult to interpret. Everything else kept constant, older migrants are healthier, which might—speculatively—suggest that in earlier migration waves mentally healthier people came to Germany from sub-Saharan Africa.

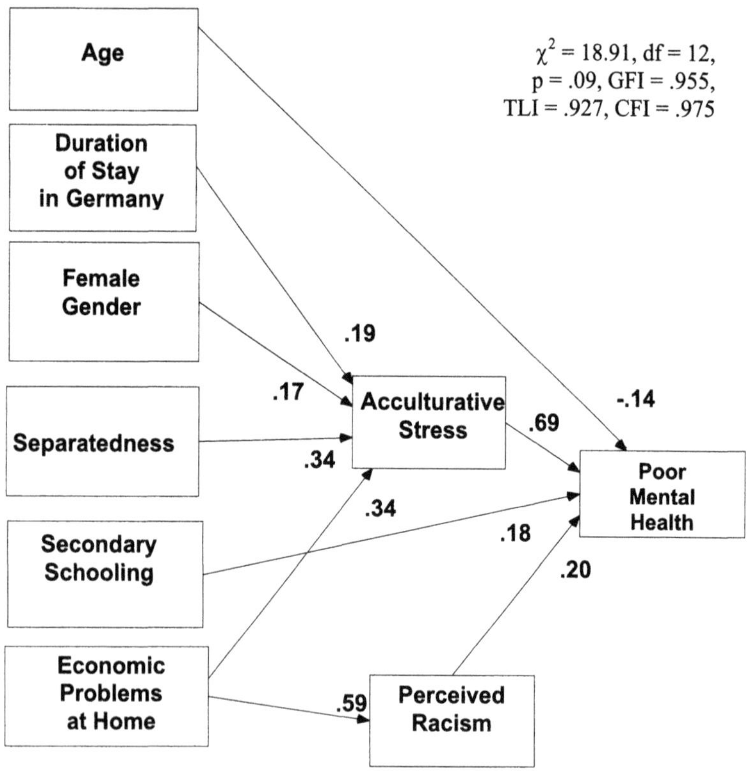

Figure 21: *Prediction of Mental Health*

Table 8
Standardized Total, Direct, and Indirect Effects in Predicting Poor Mental Health

Predictor	Total Effect	Direct Effect	Indirect Effect
Age	-.14	-.14	---
Duration of Stay in Germany	.13	---	.13
Female Gender	.12	---	.12
Separatedness	.23	---	.23
Secondary Schooling	.18	.18	---
Economic Problems at Home	.36	---	.36
Acculturative Stress	.69	.69	---
Perceived Racism	.20	.20	---

As per design of the present study, it can, of course, not be ruled out that there also is reverse causation in the way that poor mental health determines the amount of acculturative stress experienced. SEM models that test this assumption provide no better fit than the model reported in Figure 21. Furthermore, models that allow for an additional reverse path, though problematic from a statistical point of view, suggest that reverse causation is smaller than the causation direction implied by the model reported above.

In summary, we, thus, feel confident to say that those migrants who are sometimes labeled stereotypically as economic refugees (and label themselves as such, when asked for their migration motivation) have a particularly hard time to acculturate in Germany and seemingly are also the first and foremost victims of racism. The other, so-to-speak, big stressor is the difficult family-life situation African migrants find themselves in. Sizable numbers of them are separated from their spouses, be that because their spouses stayed behind or because the marriage they had in Germany did not succeed. Separatedness is the next biggest stressor after economic refugee status. German racism does have negative mental health implications, but is not as sizable in its impact as more general acculturative stressors.

10. Values, Acculturative Stress, Racism and Mental Health

In our analyses of the role of values in the interplay of acculturative stress and mental health, we first tested whether value preferences function as a moderator of the relationship between stress and health. To assume a moderating role of value preferences for this relationship means that values are assumed to affect the interrelation of the two in a way that among people with high preferences of certain values the relationship between acculturative stress and mental health is, e.g., strong, while among people with low preferences for that value it is weak. It does not seem implausible that among people with strong preferences for openness values the relationship between stress and health is weaker than among people with low preferences for such values: People who cherish openness values can be assumed to be more accepting of challenging experiences as the ones causing acculturative stress than people who have sub-average openness values. For persons accepting stressful experiences more easily, these events might then have less of an impact on mental health. For none of the four higher-order value orientations laid out in Schwartz's Theory of Values (self-transcendence. conservation, self-enhancement, and openness), however, did a moderation effect emerge.

In light of this finding we set out to inspect the role of values as predictors of acculturative stress, perceived racism, and mental health more in depth. Also in this context a few plausible assumptions can be formulated. African migrants who cherish values that are also cherished by the mainstream of the host society should experience less acculturative stress and perceive less racism. Of the four higher-order value orientations Germans tend to favor self-transcendence and openness values more than conservation and self-enhancement values. We, thus, assume that self-transcendence and openness values will go along with lower, self-enhancement and conservation values with higher degrees of acculturative stress.

As for perceived racism, hypotheses are more difficult to formulate. Here it seems plausible to assume that self-enhancement values go along with higher perceived racism, because individuals who like to put themselves through and ahead of others will more easily see hostile behavior from the vis-à-vis. As for the other three higher-order value orientations, we refrain from formulating clear assumptions, because the argumentation can soon become quite complex, when, for example, one considers whether Africans cherishing self-transcendence values will rather see Germans as holding similar or opposing convictions, racism ratings being low in the first and high in the second case.

Figure 22 reports the essence of our analyses. In it only significant paths ($p \leq .05$) from higher-order value preferences to acculturative stress, perceived racism, and (poor) mental health are documented. In the analyses we conducted, preferences of higher-order value types have been partialed for mean individual value ratings across all single value items. Higher-order value preferences have furthermore been dichotomized into high and low preferences. Intercorrelations of value preferences as well as intercorrelations of acculturative stress and perceived racism were also allowed in the tested model, but are not documented in the figure in order to not blur the plasticity of the findings.

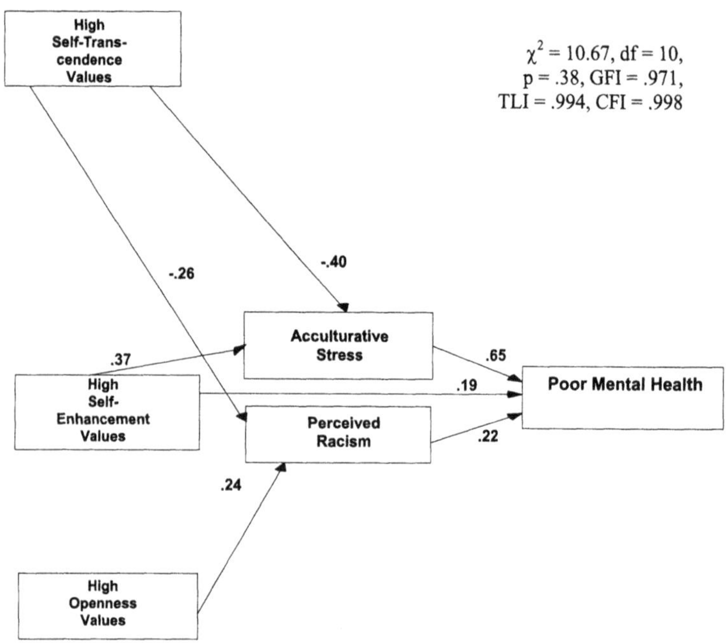

Figure 22: *Values as Predictor of Acculturative Stress, Perceived Racism, and Mental Health*

Table 8
Standardized Total, Direct, and Indirect Effects in Predicting Poor Mental Health

Predictor	Total Effect	Direct Effect	Indirect Effect
High Self-Transcendence Values	-.32	---	-.32
High Conservation Values	---	---	---
High Self-Enhancement Values	.43	.19	.23
High Openness Values	.05	---	..05
Acculturative Stress	.65	.65	---
Perceived Racism	.22	.22	---

Figure 22 and Table 8 show that value preferences indeed affect mental health: African migrants who cherish self-enhancement values (power and achievement values), which are not very popular in Germany, suffer from a poorer mental health than their fellow migrants who do not cherish these values to a high extent. Self-enhancement values are positively related both to acculturative stress and—directly—to (poor) mental health. High self-transcendence values go along with good mental health in that they are expressed by respondents who suffer less from acculturative stress. Openness and conservation values, somewhat surprisingly, had no impact on acculturative stress and only openness values predicted—higher—perceived racism scores.

In summary, one can say that individual value preferences do affect the mental health of African immigrants in Germany: Those migrants who hold values common among Germans (self-transcendence values) experience less acculturative stress than those migrants who cherish self-enhancement values which are rarely favored by Germans. Although individual acculturation strategies were not assessed in the present study, value orientations might serve as a proxy here: If migrants have adopted values commonly in high regard among Germans, they may be said to have exercised an acculturation style that nears the style Berry (1989) has labeled 'integration.' Although a comprehensive—multivariate—analysis is not possible with the present study (due to sample size restrictions), it can be said that value preferences explain as much variance in mental health as do marital status and migration motivation.

11. Discussion and Conclusions

This study investigated demographic characteristics, value preferences, perceptions of living conditions, and how these impact wellbeing among African migrants in Germany. The sample included legal and illegal residents as well as prison inmates. In spite of the fact that the sample is small in size, there is no indication that it differs in its composition from a sample that is representative in a more technical sense: All major demographic variables are reflected in adequate proportions in the sample.

The aim of the research was to provide a quantitative case study of the nature and extent of psychosocial problems African migrants encounter in Germany, based on the premise that living in Germany would be stressful for Africans more so than if they lived in an English or French, or for that matter Portuguese-speaking country, where at least the common language can serve as some sort of entry ticket. As Germany lost all its (few) African colonies already as a consequence of World War I, a common colonial history can also not serve as a familiar frame of reference for African migrants. In Germany, they are indeed what is often termed 'aliens' in legal migration lingo: Visible outsiders in a cultural context that is generally not prepared for them.

Although the design of the study is obviously not prone to offer reliable epidemiological data, the study has made it evident that African migrants in Germany are by no means in good shape health-wise and with regard to their general life circumstances. Depression, somatic and psychosomatic health problems, and psychological dysfunction including work interference seem to run particularly high. Respondents with—clinically relevant—high depression scores—probably at least a quarter of those surveyed—suffer from significant depressive thoughts, such as apathy about life, feelings of hopelessness, or thoughts of suicide. Respondents, who express strong health problems—also at least one fifth of those surveyed—suffer from serious problems across several body systems and have to cope with gastrointestinal, neurological, cardiovascular, respiratory and other conspicuous symptoms. Respondents who score high on the MMPI work interference scale—also some 20 % of all respondents—tend to have low self-confidence, concentration difficulties, obsessiveness sentiments, tension and pressure feelings, and decision making problems, which are likely to contribute to poor work performance for those who are able to find a decent job.

Acculturative stress arises predominantly from the inability to find a decent job, but also from the mere volume of daily hassles, and—not to forget—from the racial discrimination African migrants experience in Germany. Many respondents at the same time report that their economic situation and standard of living has improved substantially from the time before they migrated.

What does at first sight look like a praise of Germany is most likely constituting a major trap for Africans living in the country: Their life circumstances are far from satisfactory in absolute terms, but the fact that they are economically more bearable than they used to be in their home countries motivates them to stay. This situation has features of a double bind: If a migrant seeks a radical solution to his or her problematic situation in Germany, looking for a new migration destiny or even returning to Africa may appear as a good idea. Putting this idea into reality would then, however, typically encompass a major deterioration of one's economic situation. The knowledge that this would be the case more or less instantaneously clearly negates the option to leave the problematic situation in Germany: The African migrant finds him or herself in a vicious circle.

The present study does offer empirical evidence that Africans in Germany indeed experience this vicious circle: Their self-reported acculturative stress *increases* with the years of stay in Germany instead of decreasing with the longer adjustment time.

As the study has shown that acculturative stress is strongly related to poor mental health, one can say in all clarity that many migrants are made sicker by staying in Germany longer, but at the same time the situation in the home countries of African immigrants to Germany endangers livelihood in an existential way as well, were migrants to consider remigration.

The described vicious circle is even intensified by the fact that those migrants who came to Germany for predominantly economic reasons, i.e., those often derogatively labeled economic refugees, are the ones who are worse off. They experience the relatively highest degrees of racism and increased levels of acculturative stress, but at the same time they are the ones who have no realistic option to return to their home countries or move on to a new migration destiny.

In general terms, the results of the present study are in line with the migration-morbidity hypothesis (Klimidis & Minas, 1995; Hutchinson & Haasen, 2004) of increased risk of schizophrenia for non-white migrants in Europe, attributed to social inequalities, family fragmentation, and migratory stress.

Family fragmentation was indeed one of the problems that impacted mental health of African migrants most: Migrants who reported to be separated from their spouses (for whatever reason), were at the same time the one's who reported highest levels of acculturative stress. It should be emphasized that the present study clearly showed that family fragmentation is not a direct predictor of poor mental health but predicts increased levels of acculturative stress, which in turn predict poor mental health. Such a result supports the argumentation that the connection between family fragmentation and poor mental health is *not* based on a selection process. It is not the people whose family is fragmented already at home who then leave their home country to seek their luck abroad. Such an explanation would only be plausible if separatedness would at least in part also serve as a direct predictor of poor mental health. The effect of separatedness on mental health is, however, completely mediated by acculturative stress. Migration 'socializes' separation, which in turn increases acculturative stress and consequentially poor mental health.

Fernando (1993) has claimed that racism is the most serious risk factor for African immigrants to Western and in that sense 'white' countries. This claim is not fully supported in the present study; other stressors seem to make a stronger impact, but perceived racism is a non-negligible source of poor mental health as well. So, our findings are also in line with findings by Ataca (1996), Furnham and Shiekh (1993), Vega, Gil, Warheit, Zimmerman, and Apospori (1993), and Ward and Chang (1997), who have reported negative correlations of perceived discrimination or prejudice and psychological wellbeing.

Tanaka, Takai, Kohyama, and Fujihara (1994) as well as Ward and Searle, (1991) have argued in more general terms that attitudes held by members of the dominant culture strongly influence patterns of immigrant adaptation. This is presumably not just the case in a somehow passive way, a way that makes migrants the victims, for example, of racism in cases where racism is a common phenomenon in the host society. Attitudes and values prevalent in the host society also serve as a frame for acculturation strategies of immigrants. Immigrants ignorant of attitudes and values of the host society will have a much harder time to acculturate, and will experience more acculturative stress than immigrants who are sensitive to the prevailing values and beliefs of the host society. Ward, Bochner and Furnham (2001) have argued that values, as evaluative beliefs, are cognitive constructs tied to self-definition. For African immigrants to Germany this may mean that values are one of the few accessible entry tickets into German society. Of the four acculturation orientations described by Berry (1989; Sam & Berry, 1995, 2006), assimilation, integration, separation, and marginalization, assimilation is likely to have the lowest a priori probability, because Blacks in Germany will obviously have great difficulties to assimilate to Germans for 'natural' reasons. They cannot realistically give up their African or Black identity, because they will remain members of a visible minority for multiple generations. For the same reason, marginalization is also not a highly likely acculturation orientation, a priori, because members of visible minorities will also have less of a chance to flee their cultural community of upbringing. This special case of African migrants in a 'white,' Western context then leaves them with the option of resorting to a separation or an integration orientation. Separation would mean that they remain only in the cultural context of Africans in Germany. Integration would mean that they retain their African identity, while at the same time becoming open for 'German-ness.' We argue that adopting values prevalent in the German society is a viable way towards an integration orientation to acculturation. Our study shows that those African immigrants to Germany who hold above-average self-transcendence values (universalism, benevolence), experience significantly less acculturative stress than migrants who cherish self-enhancement values (power, achievement). They even see themselves as victims of racism less frequently. Immigrants who cherish power values, hierarchy values from a culture-level perspective, which are in no way cherished in Germany, do experience more acculturative stress and even report a poorer mental health that is not mediated by acculturative stress.

To round up our conclusions to be drawn from the study we conducted, we will finally relate our findings to the most prominent theoretical concepts offered in the field of acculturation consequences, as we had spelt them out in the introduction of the present volume. Some verbatim citations from these earlier sections will become obvious in our attempt to link our findings to earlier scientific endeavors in the field.

To explain the psychological aspects of migration and inter-culture contact, several theoretical frameworks have been forwarded to explain how stress is experienced.

The stress-and-coping framework (Ward, Bochner, & Furnham, 2001) assumes that because the experience of intercultural contact and change occurs in a socio-political and economic context and is influenced by the characteristics of the migrant's society of origin and society of settlement, changes associated with inter-culture contact are precipitating stress which results in affective, behavioral and cognitive coping responses. Here our study results imply that African immigrants in Germany seemingly do not have very successful coping strategies at hand. This can be drawn from the fact that the self-reported degree of acculturative stress determines a migrant's mental health status to almost 50 %. Would coping strategies be more successful this percentage can be expected to be considerably lower. Readers should note that such a summary does not suggest that non-successful coping with acculturative stress in large segments of the African migrant community in Germany is the 'fault' of the individual migrant. German racism and the difficult legal situation of many African migrants have their share in limiting the degrees of freedom of African migrants in choosing appropriate strategies for coping with acculturative stress.

The Similarity-Attraction Hypothesis (Byrne, 1969) also presupposes that Africans and Germans are different on idiosyncratic characteristics, which will therefore lead to stereotypes (Social Categorization Theory) and consequently racial discrimination. This assumption does find some support in that racial discrimination indeed adds to poor mental health, but the 'effect size' associated with racism as a source of poor mental health is small, but by no means negligible.

As for gender differences, our supposition that male migrants, often being the more overt victims of racism, should exhibit worse mental health scores was not corroborated. It emerged that women experienced more acculturative stress and consequentially a poorer mental health, particularly as pertaining to depression and work interference, but also with regard to treatment resistance.

These results support the differential vulnerability hypothesis, differential exposure hypothesis, and social role theory. The differential vulnerability hypothesis assumes that given exposure to similar life stresses and strains, women are more likely than men to manifest symptoms of psychopathology. The hypothesis focuses on both contextual factors and features of feminine socialization that may render women more inclined than men to react to life difficulties with feelings of self-blame and a sense of helplessness and hopelessness (Brown & Harris, 1978; Makosky, 1982). The hypothesis on differential exposure focuses on the role that various work-related strains play in contributing to excess levels of psychopathology among women in general and married women in particular (Aneshensel, Frerichs & Clark 1981, Cleary & Mechanic, 1983).

However, the work of Makosky (1980, 1982) and Greywolf, Ashlay, and Reese (1982) raises questions as to whether such strains are the most salient risk factors for depression in the lives of women. These authors emphasize the etiological significance of a very different set of life strains such as the absence of a spouse, social isolation, chronic poverty, and poor health, all of which involve major resources deficits that have been linked to depression, (Warheit, 1975). Our study supports this explanation in one result in particular: It is divorced women who report the highest levels of acculturative stress, separated women reporting the second highest level of stress, married women still a somewhat high level, and only single women a low level of stress. Among men, the picture is dramatically different. Divorced men report lowest levels of stress with single and married men reporting similarly low levels. Only among separated men levels of acculturative stress are higher then among women from the same marital status group. This finding suggests that being divorced as well as being married 'means' something different for women and men: A divorced man is 'free' again and can put his energies into coping with the tasks of acculturation; he seemingly does not experience high amounts of stress, because 'his hands are free' for adequate coping, as he no longer has to perform the roles of head of family and bread winner. A divorced woman, but also a married woman, on the other hand, seems to have to bear the chores of social isolation and the shame of being divorced (divorcees) and of double responsibilities for husband/family and on the job (married women). This situation leaves woman with fewer resources for coping with acculturation tasks.

Although social role theory is frequently referred to as a gender role theory (e.g., Rosenfield, 1980), the explanatory framework developed by Gove and Tudor (1973) clearly invokes gender-specific social roles—wife/husband, mother/father, housewife/worker—rather than the global male and female distinction to account for gender differences in mental illness. Gove (1972) specifically claimed that it is the roles that women occupy, rather than some characteristics of women's generalized sex role, which make women more susceptible to mental illness. A key explanatory element in this orientation in the purported greater stress placed on married women, as compared with that placed on married men or the unmarried of both sexes, by extensive familiar role demands. Inferences drawn from the results of the present study suggest that indeed this seems to be the case.

However, older studies concerning social roles have shown mixed results. Radloff (1978) reports that marital status, employment status, and sex interact in their relationship to mental illness, but concludes that these social roles are inadequate to account for gender differences in mental illness. Fox (1980) presented results of three different national studies of untreated mental illness, which indicate that women are more likely to be mentally ill than men regardless of marital status. Here our study obviously speaks a different language: Divorce and separation in particular, but to some degree even marriage predict acculturative stress and consequentially poor mental health differentially among men and women.

Cross-border movement is as old as history can recall. It goes back to times when borders were markers of territories of different quality and not legal frontiers. Current trends of African youths moving to western societies are, however, unprecedented. Many African youths believe that to put an end to ones problem is to travel to Europe and the North Americas thinking that it is all bed of roses, 'lands flowing with milk and honey.' So they travel in droves and many travel by extremely unsafe means. Some trek through the 'valleys and shadows of death' of the hot Sahara desert, trolleys, dinghy and cargo ships. On arrival many find that the land that was supposed to flow with milk and honey actually flows with racism, hardships, imprisonment, police harassments, daily apprehension of deportation, and other hosts of hostile life situations. Coping life styles are then channeled into drug trade (a common sight at the *Hauptbahnhof* in larger German cities), prostitution, and domestic thefts, and as a result, non-negligible numbers then find their homes in prisons, lockouts, asylums, and mental institutions.

The present study can be summarized as having corroborated the following facts:

- A majority of Africans in Germany reported their present situation in Germany as being negative.
- A precarious job, a huge volume of daily hassles, and racial discrimination were singled out as the predominant problems experienced in Germany.
- Acculturative stress and perceived racism significantly affected mental health, first and foremost fostering depression, somatic and psychosomatic health problems, and psychological dysfunction interfering with one's work performance.
- Woman experienced more acculturative stress and consequentially a poorer mental health, particularly with regard to depression, work interference problems, and therapy resistance.
- Acculturative stress increased with the duration of stay in Germany

- Family fragmentation, in general, and being separated from one's spouse, in particular, is one of the strongest predictor of acculturative stress
- Among all African migrants those who have come as 'economic refugees' are the ones worse off.
- Having had only little education at home (lower level secondary) constitutes a risk factor for African migrants.
- Prison inmates differ from members of the general population of African migrants only to a marginal extent.
- Holding value preferences in line with value preferences prevalent in the German societal mainstream serves as a buffer against acculturative stress.

12. Impact, Consequences and Recommendations

Migration experts have argued that the contribution of the developing world to the developed is relatively marginal. When people emigrate, it may ease shortages of the labor market in the target countries, but it will at the same time constitute a serious brain drain for the sending countries (Pillay, 2007).

Others argue that international migration encourages economic development and benefits both sending and receiving countries. Obviously, developed economies benefit by improving their global competitiveness through importing both the skilled and unskilled labor they need (van Dijkhorst & Hilhorst, 2006).

Another view is that in Africa's stagnating and deteriorating economies, emigration contributes to development by relieving unemployment and providing remittances from abroad that increase the supply of needed foreign exchange. It is pointed that the flows between African and developed countries do not go just one way. Africa is also the recipient of highly skilled labor migrants from developed countries from such sources as the Peace Corps, USAID, the World Bank, the UN, and staff of multinational corporations (Gupta, Pattillo, & Wagh, 2009).

While there are unresolved debates about, the positive and negative effects of remittances on countries of emigration, it is clear that remittances from international migration are sizeable and important sources of foreign exchange. Although the poorest seldom have the means to migrate, remittances have been shown to play an important role in poverty alleviation from migrant households and in sub-national areas of out-migration. The consequences of remittances for income inequality depend greatly on the income composition of a given migrant stream.

The problems of migration are complex. The complexity of Africans migrating to Western societies is anchored on person-attitudinal and country-problem variables. The person-attitudinal variable is a problem among African youths who believe that travelling to first world nations is an end in itself for greener pasture and putting an end to their economic woes. But how true is this belief system to real life experiences in Europe and the Americas? On the country-problem variables, why do migrants run away from their home countries and what are African countries and their leaders doing about this in terms of prevention by creating jobs for the youths, avoid wars etc. How can African Union (AU) help in this regard? What about the roles of Continental Europe and America and various host countries? How is international politics helping to aggravate the problem of poverty in African countries and finding solutions to the problems?

As earlier said, the situation is complex and demands multifaceted solutions and these should include broadly: Attitudinal change among youths in Africa. Such behavior change program should target real life experiences among migrants in developed nations for youths who believe that western countries flow with milk and honey.

African Governments particularly those where emigrations are common (West, East and some Southern African countries) should expedite economic and social action reforms in their countries to minimize the need to migrate.

Host countries should put in place humane programs to minimize triggering factors that can predispose migrants to psychological problems. These programs should also target the local population on developing positive attitude to migrants.

In addition, psychological practices in host countries should begin to seriously recognize the role of cross-cultural factors in mental health including attributions of illness, diagnoses, and treatment.

The results of this study emphasize the importance and nature of racial problems experienced by African migrants in Germany. But not only anti-racism programs are high on the German agenda. Demand-tailored counseling offers for Africans in Germany and genuine attempts to support family cohesion and family reunion are at least of equal importance. An unofficial attitude of "you should not be here in the first place" has a negative impact not only on the migrants, but is at the same time costly for Germany in that it is prone to increase the need to allocate more incarceration places, more emergency medical care, more administrative and police personnel: The welcomed immigrant is the cheaper immigrant! The study showed a majority of unhappy people faced with racial discrimination and no decent jobs even when they are qualified but yet cannot go back home because social, economic and political situations are worse in their home countries.

To sum up, we may cautiously suppose that many of the challenges (trafficking and illegal routing, migrant rights and integration, education/information for citizens of receiving and sending countries) be carefully appraised and studies pursued in this direction as the world continues to globalize.

According to Chimanikire (2004), there are two related factors that will determine the scale of future African immigration to developed countries. (1) Economic and political developments in Africa and (2) Policies on immigration and refugees of the developed countries.

According to Chimanikire (2002, p. 22), "it can be maintained that the best antidote to migration from the Third World and from Africa in particular is helping poor countries achieve more peaceful societies, freer and more democratic political systems, and higher economic growth. This would necessitate in many cases higher levels of aid and investment from the rich, industrial nations so alarmed by the influx of unwanted immigrants. As long as the global economy continues to mainly benefit the already rich, many people in stagnant, politically unstable Third World countries will continue to have no recourse but to emigrate, illegally if not legally. There is a large and growing pool of African scientists living and working in the industrialized world. While Asian (e.g. India) countries have developed and adopted strategies to mobilize and utilize their Diaspora, African countries lack such measures. The region can no longer afford to ignore this capital. Indeed it should tap the enormous scientific and technological talents of Africans abroad and use them for its own scientific and technological development."

References

Abrams, D. & Hogg, M. A. (Eds.) (1990). *Social identity theory: Constructive and critical advances*. London: Harvester Wheatsheaf.

Adepoju, A. (1992) Migrant Africa. *Unesco Courier, 45* (1), 36-39.

Aneshensel, C. S., Frerichs, R. R., & Clark, V. A. (1981). Family roles and sex differences in depression. *Journal of Health and Social Behaviour, 22,* 379-393.

Ataca, B. (1996). *Psychological and sociocultural adaptation of Turkish immigrants, Canadians, and Turks.* Paper presented at the 13th Congress of International Association for Cross-Cultural Psychology, Montreal, Canada, July.

Aycan, Z. & Berry, J. W. (1996). Impact of employment-related experiences on Turkish immigrants' psychological well-being and adaptation to Canada. *Canadian Journal of Behavioural Science, 28*, 240-251.

Babiker, I. E., Cox, J. L., & Miller, P. (1980). The measurement of cultural distance and its relationship to medical consultation, symptomatology, and examination performance of overseas students at Edinburgh University. *Social Psychiatry, 15*, 109-116.

Beck, A. & Greenberg, R. (1974). Cognitive therapy with depressed women. In F. Violet & B. Vasanti (Eds.), *Women in Therapy* (pp. 113-131). New York: Brunner-Mazel.

Berner, C. H. (1998) *Standardisation of the Minnesota Multiphasic Personality Inventory-2: Content and validity scales in the Yoruba Population of the Ibadan region.* University of Ibadan: Unpublished PhD Thesis.

Berry, J. W. (1989). Acculturation and psychological adaptation. In J. P. Forgas and J. M. Innes (Eds.), *Recent advances in social psychology: An international perspective* (pp. 511-520). Amsterdam: Elsevier.

Berry, J. W. (1997). Immigration, acculturation and adaptation. *Applied Psychology and International Review, 46*, 5-36.

Berry, J. W. (2005). Acculturation: Living successfully in two cultures. *International Journal of Intercultural Relations, 29*, 697-712.

Berry, J.W. (2006). Stress perspectives on acculturation. In D. Sam & J. W. Berry, (Eds.) *Cambridge handbook of acculturation psychology* (pp. 43-57). Cambridge: Cambridge University Press

Blackford, J., Street, A., & Parsons, C. (1997). Breaking down language barriers in clinical practice. *Contemporary Nurse, 6,* 15-21.

Bochner, S. & Cairns, L. G. (1976). An unobtrusive measure of helping behaviour toward aborigines. In G. E. Kearney & D. W. McElwain (Eds.), *Aboriginal condition: Retrospect and prospec*t (pp. 344–356). Canberra: Australian Institute of Aboriginal Studies.

Boswell, C. & Crisp, J. (2004). *Poverty, international migration and asylum.* Helsinki, United Nations University, World Institute for Development Economics Research.

Brown, W. & Harris, T. (1978). *Social origins of depression: A study of psychiatric disorder in women.* New York: Free Press.

Byrne, D. (1969). Attitudes and attraction. *Advances in the experimental social psychology, 4,* 35-89.

Chimanikire, D. P. (2002). *African migration: causes, consequences and future prospects and policy options.* Paper presented at the United Nations University/World Institute for Development Economics Research Conference "Poverty, International Migration, and Asylum," Helsinki, September.

Chimanikire, D. P. (2004). *Plight of children in conflict and post–conflict societies: The case of Africa.* Paper presented at the United Nations University/World Institute for Development Economics Research Conference "Making Peace Work," Helsinki, June.

Cleary, P. O. & Mechanic, D. (1983). Sex differences and psychological distress among married people. *Journal of Health and Social Behaviour, 24*, 111-121.

Cohrs, J. C., Moschner, B., Maes, J., & Kielmann, S. (2005). The motivational bases of right-wing authoritarianism and social dominance orientation: Relations to values and attitudes in the aftermath of September 11, 2001. *Personality and Social Psychology Bulletin, 31*, 1425-1434.

Comino, E., Silove, D., Manicavasagar, V., Harris, E., & Harris, M. (2001). Agreement in symptoms of anxiety and depression between patients and GPs: the influence of ethnicity. *Family Practice, 18*, 71-77.

Deaux, K. (1976). *The behaviour of women and men.* Monterey, CA: Brooks/Cole.

European Union (2005). *Common basic principles for immigrant integration policy in the European Union*. Brussels: European Commission.

Fernando, S. (1993). Racism and Xenophobia. *Innovation of Social Science Research, 6,* 9-19.

Fox, J. W. (1980). Gove's specific sex role theory of mental illness: A research note. *Journal of Health and Social Behaviour, 21*, 260-267.

Frank-Bosch, B. (2002). Verdienstabstand zwischen Männern und Frauen. Eine Untersuchung mit Hilfe der laufenden Verdiensterhebungen 2001. *Wirtschaft und Statistik, 5*, 395-409.

Furnham, A. & Shiekh, S. (1993). Gender, generational and social support correlates of mental health in Asian immigrants. *International Journal of Social Psychiatry, 39*, 22-33.

Gorman, D., Brough M., & Ramirez E. (2003). How young people from culturally and linguistically diverse backgrounds experience mental health: Some insights for mental health nurses. *International Journal of Mental Health Nursing, 12*, 194-202.

Gove, W. R. (1972). The relationship between sex roles, marital status and mental illness. *Social Forces, 51*, 34-44.

Gove, W. R. & Tudor, J. F. (1973). Adult sex roles and mental illness. *American Journal of Sociology, 78* (4), 812-835.

Greywolf, E., Ashlay, D., & Reese, M. F. (1982). Physical health issues. In D. Belle (Ed.). *Lives in Stress: Women and Depression* (pp. 211f.). Beverly Hills: Sage Publications.

Gupta, S., Pattillo, C., & Wagh, S. (2009). Effect of remittances on poverty and financial development in sub-Saharan Africa. *World Development, 37*, 104-115.

Hathaway, S. R. (1960). *An MMPI Handbook* (Vol. 1). Minneapolis: University of Minnesota Press.

Hathaway, S. R. & McKinley, J. C. (1943). *Manual for the Minnesota Multiphasic Personality Inventory*. New York: Psychological Corporation.

Helmes, E. & Reddon, J.R. (1993). A perspective on development in assessing psychopathology: A critical review of the MMPI and MMPI-2. *Psychological Bulletin, 113*, 453-471.

Holbrook, A., Krosnick, J. A., & Pfent, A. M. (2007). Response rates in surveys by the news media and government contractor survey research firms. In J. Lepkowski, N. C. Tucker, J. M. Brick, E. D. de Leeuw, L. Japec, P. J. Lavrakas, M. W. Link, & R. L. Sangster (Eds.), *Advances in Telephone Survey Methodology* (pp. 499-528). New York: Wiley.

Hutchinson, G. & Haasen, C. (2004). Migration and schizophrenia: the challenges for European psychiatry and implications for the future. *Social Psychiatry and Psychiatric Epidemiology, 39* (5), 350-357.

Idemudia, E. S. (2005). African migrants in Germany: A psychological perspective. Bremen: Report to the Alexander von Humboldt Foundation.

Idemudia, E. S. (2006). Global movement and health potential of black migrants in Germany: A study of mental health indices using MMPI. In TRANS. Internet-Zeitschrift für Kulturwissenschaften. No.16/2005 [http://www.inst.at/trans/16Nr/08_3/idemudia16.htm].

Idemudia, E. S. & Boehnke K. (2005). Globalisierung, Afrika und afrikanische Immigranten in Deutschland: Ein empirischer Bericht. In A. Groh (Ed.) *be-WEG-ung: Akademische Perspektiven auf Reisen und Ortswechsel* (pp. 49-69). Berlin: Weidler.

Idemudia, E. S., & Boehnke, K. (2006). An assessment of african migrants' attitude in Germany: Implication for international migration, intercultural contact, and globalization. *Psychopathologie Africaine, 32*, 5-20.

Jagodzinski, W. & Greeley, A. (1998). *The demand for religion: Hard core atheism and 'supply side' theory*. Chicago: unpublished manuscript [http://www.agreeley.com/articles/hardcore.html].

Katz, D. & Braly, K. (1933). Racial stereotypes of one hundred college students. *Journal of Abnormal and Social Psychology, 28,* 280-290.

Kessler, R. C. & McLeod, J. W. (1984). Sex differences in vulnerability to undesirable life events. *American Sociological Review, 49*, 620-631.

Ki-Zerbo, J. (2003). *A quand l'Afrique?* Paris: Éditions de l'Aube.

Klimidis, S. & Minas, H. (1995). Migration, culture, and mental health in children and adolescents. In C. Guerra & R. White (Eds.), *Ethnic minority youth in Australia* (pp. 85-100). Hobart: National Clearinghouse for Youth Studies.

Lambert, J. R. (1971). *Crime, Police and Race Relations*. Oxford: Oxford University Press.

Lippman, W. (1922). *Public opinion*. New York: Hartcourt & Brace.

Littlewood R. & Lipsedge, M. (1989) *Aliens and alienists: Ethnic minorities and psychiatry*. London: Unwin Hyman Ltd.

Logiudice, D., Hassett, A., Cook, R., Flicker, L., & Ames, D. (2001). Equity of access to a memory clinic in Melbourne? Non-English speaking background attenders are more severely demented and have increased rates of psychiatric disorders. *International Journal of Geriatric Psychiatry, 16,* 327-334.

Makosky, V. P. (1980). Stress and the mental health of women: A discussion of research and issues. In M. Guttentag, D. Salasin, & D. Belle (Eds.), *The mental health of women* (pp. 111-128). New York: Academy Press.

Makosky, V. P. (1982). Sources of stress: Events or conditions. In D. Belle (Ed.), *Lives in stress: Women and depression* (pp. 35-53). Beverly Hills: Sage.

Marshall G. (1994). *The concise Oxford dictionary of sociology*. Oxford: Oxford University Press.

Martin, P. (2002). *Economic integration and migration: The Mexico-US case*. Paper presented at the United Nations University/World Institute for Development Economics Research Conference "Poverty, International Migration, and Asylum," Helsinki, September.

Myers, D. G. (1995). *Psychology*. New York: Worth Publishers.

Newmann, J. P. (1982). *Sex differences in depression: A test of alternative explanations for the greater vulnerability of women to depression*. Madison: University of Wisconsin, unpublished PhD Thesis.

Newmark, C. S. & McCord, D. M. (1996). The Minnesota Multiphasic Personality Inventory-2 (MMPI-2). In C. S. Newmark (Ed.), *Major psychological assessment instruments* (pp. 1-58). Boston: Allyn and Bacon.

Opitz, M., Oguntoye, K., & Schultz, D. (1992). *Showing our colors: Afro-German women speak out.* Amherst: The University of Massachusetts Press.

Pillay, R. (2007). A conceptual framework for the strategic analysis and management of the brain drain of African health care professionals. *African Journal of Business Management, 1*, 26-33.

Radloff, L. S. (1978). Sex differences in depression: The effects of occupation and marital status. *Sex Roles, 1,* 249-265.

Radloff, L. S. & Monroe, M. K. (1978). Sex differences in helplessness with implication for depression. In L. S. Hansen & R. S. Rapesa (Eds.). *Career development and counseling of women* (pp. 199-221). Springfield, Illinois: Charles C. Thomas.

Radloff, L. S., & Rae, D. S. (1981). Components of the sex differences in depression. In R. G. Simmons (Ed.), *Research in Community and Mental Health* (pp. 77-110). Greenwich, CT: JAI.

Rosenfield, S. (1980). Sex differences in depression: Do women always have higher status? *Journal of Health and Social Behaviour, 21*, 33-42.

Sam, D. L. & Berry, J. W. (1995). Acculturative stress among young immigrants in Norway. *Scandinavian Journal of Psychology, 36*, 240-253.

Sam, D. L. & Berry, J. W. (Eds.) (2006). *Cambridge handbook of acculturation psychology.* Cambridge: Cambridge University Press.

Schwartz, S. H. (1992). Universals in the content and structure of values: Theoretical advances and empirical tests in 20 countries. *Advances in Experimental Social Psychology,* 25, 1-65.

Schwartz, S. H. (1994). Are there universal aspects in the structure and contents of human values? *Journal of Social Issues, 50*, 19-45.

Schwartz, S. H., Melech, G., Lehmann, A., Burgess, S., Harris, M., & Owens, V. (2001). Extending the cross-cultural validity of the theory of basic human values with a different method of measurement. *Journal of Cross-Cultural Psychology, 32*, 519-542.

Schwartz, S. H. & Sagiv, L. (1995). Identifying culture-specifics in the content and structure of values. *Journal of Cross-Cultural Psychology, 26,* 92-116.

Seligman, M. E. P. (1975). *Helplessness on depression, development and death.* San Francisco: W.N. Freeman.

Tajfel, H. (1970). Experiments in intergroup discrimination. *Scientific American, 223,* 92-102.

Tajfel, H. (1981). *Human groups and social categories.* Cambridge: Cambridge University Press.

Tanaka, T., Takai, J., Kohyama, T. & Fujihara, T. (1994). Adjustment patterns of international students in Japan. *International Journal of Intercultural Relations, 18*, 55-75.

Triandis, H. C. (1990). Theoretical concepts that are applicable to the analysis of ethnocentrism. In R. W. Brislin (Ed.), *Applied cross-cultural psychology* (pp. 34-55). Newbury Park, CA: Sage.

van Dijkhorst, H. & Hilhorst, D. (2006). Reviewing the World. *Development and Change, 37* (6), 1435-1443. Vega, W. A., Gil. A.G., Warheit, G. J., Zimmerman, R. S., & Apospori, E. (1993). Acculturation and delinquent behaviour among Cuban-American adolescents. *American Journal of Community Psychology, 21*, 113-125.

Ward, C., Bochner, S., & Furnham, A. (2001). *The Psychology of Culture Shock.* (2nd ed.). London, GB: Routledge.

Ward, C. & Chang, W. C. (1997). "Cultural fit:" A new perspective on personality and sojourner adjustment. *International Journal of Intercultural Relations, 21*, 525-533.

Ward, C. & Searle, W. (1991). The impact of value discrepancies and cultural identity on psychological and sociocultural adjustment of sojourners. *International Journal of Intercultural Relations, 15*, 209–225.

Warheit, J. (1975). Life events, coping, with stress and depressive sympthomatology. *American Journal of Psychiatry, 136*, 502-507.

Weissman, M. M. & Klerman, G. L. (1977). Sex differences and the epidemiology of depression. *Archives of General Psychiatry, 34*, 38-111.

Zuckerman, P. (2007). Atheism: Contemporary Rates and Patterns. In M. Martin (Ed.), *The Cambridge Companion to Atheism* (pp. 47-64). Cambridge: Cambridge University Press.

Appendix

Original Questionnaire Used for the Study[13]

Questionnaire Booklet

Good Morning, (Afternoon). This is a research project. We are working on a study on the needs, social values and general state of life of Africans in Germany. We are asking a sample of Africans living in Bremen to help us with answering some questions about themselves and their views on some relevant issues here in Germany. The answers you give will be used only in combination with those of other people. We will not make your individual views known to anybody. Your help in answering the questions as you personally feel will be appreciated. Your names or identity are not required.

[13] The original questionnaire has been reformatted to fit the layout of the current volume, and the meanwhile outdated contact information for the first author has been purged, but no other changes were undertaken.

Section A

Sex male ( ) female ( )

Marital status: single ( )

married & divorced ( )

married & separated ( )

married ( )

Age (in years) please state ....

Educational level before coming here (Please specify) ....

Educational level after coming here (Please specify) ....

Highest educational level (Please specify) ....

Length of stay in Germany (Specify in years) ....

Where do you come from in Africa ....

Present occupation (Specify) ....

Please in a sentence what was the reason for leaving home!

....

....

....

....

How would you describe your present experiences here in Germany?

....

....

....

Have you ever had any problem with the law? Yes ( ) No ( )

If yes, nature of problem ....

Identify problems you encounter here in Germany!

....

....

....

Section B

Please circle or tick (√) the answer that applies to you best. Ensure to answer all the questions.

		Yes	No
3	I wake up fresh and rested most mornings		
6	My father is a good man or (if your father is dead) my father was a good man		
9	My daily life is full of things that keep me interested		
10	I am about as able to work as I ever was		
11	There seems to be a lump in my throat most of the times		
12	My sex life is satisfactory		
15	I work under a great deal of tension		
16	Once in a while I think of things too bad to talk about		
17	I am sure I get a raw deal from life		
18	I am troubled by attacks of nausea and vomiting		
20	I am very seldom troubled by constipation		
21	At times I have very much wanted to leave home		
22	No one seems to understand me		
24	Evil spirits possess me at times		
25	I feel that it is certainly best to keep my mouth shut when I am in trouble		
28	I am bothered by an upset stomach several times a week		
29	At times I feel like swearing		

30	I have nightmares every few nights		
31	I find it hard to keep my mind on a task or job		
32	I have had very peculiar and strange experiences		
33	I seldom worry about my health		
35	Sometimes when I was young I stole things		
36	I have a cough most of the time		
38	I have had periods of days weeks or month when I couldn't get myself in the right mood		
39	My sleep Is fitful and disturbed		
40	Much of the times my head seems to hurt all over		
41	I do not always tell the truth		
42	If people had not had it in for me, I would have been much more successful		
44	Once a week or oftener I suddenly feel hot all over for no real reason		
45	I am in just as good physical health as much of my friends		
46	I prefer to pass by school friends or people I know but I have not seen for a long time unless they speak to me first		
47	I am almost never bothered by pains over my heart or in my chest		
48	Most anytime I would rather sit and daydream than do anything else		
49	I am a very sociable person		
51	I do not read every editorial in the news paper everyday		
52	I have not lived the right kind of life		

53	Parts of my body often have feelings like burning, tingling crawling or going to sleep		
54	My family does not like the work I have chosen. (Or the work I intend to choose for my lifework)		
56	I wish I could be as happy as other people		
57	I hardly ever feel pain in the back of my neck		
59	I am troubled by discomfort in the pith of my stomach every few days or oftener		
60	When I am with people I am bothered by hearing very strange things		
61	I am an important person		
65	Most of the time I feel unhappy		
65	It would be better if almost all laws were thrown away		
71	These days I find it hard not to give up hope of amounting to something		
72	My soul sometimes leaves my body		
73	I am certainly lacking in self confidence		
75	I usually feel like life is worthwhile		
77	Once in a while I put of until tomorrow what I can do today		
78	I am liked by most people who know me		
82	I do many things which I regret afterwards (I regret things more than others seem to do)		
83	I have very few quarrels with members of my family		
84	I was suspended form school one or more times for bad behaviour		

86	I like to go to parties and those affairs where there is lots of loud fun		
90	I love my father (or if your father is dead) I laved my father		
91	I have little or no trouble with my muscles twitching or jumping		
92	I don't seem to care what happens to me		
93	Sometimes when I am not feeling well I am easily upset		
95	I am happy most of the time		
96	I see things or animals or people around me that others do not see		
97	There seems to be a fullness in my head or most of the time		
98	Some people are so bossy that I feel like doing opposite of what they request even when I know they are right		
101	Often I feel as if there is a tight band around my head		
102	I get angry sometimes		
105	In school I was sometimes sent to the principal for bad behaviour		
107	My table manners are not quite as good at home as when I am out in company		
108	Any one who is willing and able to wok hard has a good chance of succeeding in life		
109	I seem to be as capable and smart as most others around me		
111	I have a great deal of stomach trouble		
114	Sometimes I am so strongly attracted by the personal articles		

116	Often I cant understand why I have been so upset and angry		
117	I have never vomited blood or coughed up blood		
118	I do not worry about catching diseases		
120	I frequently find it necessary to stand up for what I believe in		
122	At times my thought have raced ahead faster than I could speak them		
123	If I could get into a movie without paying and be sure I was not seen I would probably do it.		
125	I believe that my home life is as pleasant as most people I know		
126	I believe in law enforcement		
127	Criticism or scolding hurts me terribly		
130	I certainly feel useless at times		
132	I believe in a life hereafter		
134	At times I feel like picking a fist fight with somebody		
138	I believe that I am being plotted against		
139	I would rather win than loose in a game		
140	Most nights I go to sleep without thoughts or ideas bothering me		
141	During the past few years I have been well most of the times		
142	I have never had a fit or convulsion		
144	I believe I am been followed		
145	I feel that I am often punished without a cause		

146	I cry easily		
148	I have never felt better in my life than I do now		
149	The top of my head sometimes feel tender		
150	Sometimes I feel like I must injure either myself or someone else		
153	I like to know some important people because it makes me feel important		
156	I am never happy unless I am roaming or travelling around		
157	What others think of me does not bother me		
158	It makes me uncomfortable to put on a stunt at a party even when others are doing the same sort of things		
159	I have never had a fainting spell		
162	Someone has been trying to poison me		
167	I find it hard to talk when I meet people		
168	I have had periods in which I carried out activities without knowing later what I had been doing		
170	I am afraid of loosing my mind		
171	I am against giving money to beggars		
174	I like to study and read about things that I am working at		
175	I feel weak all over most of the times		
176	I have very few headaches		
179	I have had no difficulties in keeping my balance in walking		
180	There is something wrong with my mind		

181	I do not have spells of hay fever or asthma		
183	I do not like everyone I know		
184	I daydream very little		
185	I wish I were not so shy		
190	My people treat me more like a child than a grown up		
192	My mother is a god woman (or if your mother is dead) My mother was a good woman		
194	I have never had any breaking out on my skin that would harm me		
195	There is very little love and companionship in my family as in others		
198	I often hear voices without knowing where they come from		
203	I gossip a little at times		
204	My hearing is as good as most people		
205	Some of my family have habits that bother and annoy me very much		
208	I hardly ever notice my heart pounding and I am seldom short of breath		
210	I like to visit places where I have never been before		
213	I get mad easily and the get over it soon.		
215	I worry a great deal.		
216	Someone has been trying to rob me.		
217	My relatives are nearly in sympathy with me.		
222	Children should be taught all the main facts of sex.		

223	I believe that I am no more nervous most people.		
224	I have few or no pains.		
227	I don't blame people for trying to grab everything they cat get in this world.		
228	There are persons who are trying to steal my thoughts and ideas.		
232	Sometime in elections I vote for people about whom I know very little.		
233	I have difficulty in starting to do tings.		
234	I believe I am a condemned person.		
235	I was a slow learner in school.		
240	At time it has been impossible for me to keep from stealing or shoplifting something.		
243	When in a group of people I have trouble thinking of the right thing to talk about.		
246	I believe my sins are unpardonable.		
247	I have numbness in one or more places of my skin.		
248	I do not blame people for taking advantage of people who leave themselves open to it.		
249	My eye is as good as it has been for years.		
250	At times I have been so entertained by cleverness of some criminals that have hoped they would of get away with it.		
252	Everything tastes the same.		
255	I do not often notice my ears ringing or buzzing.		
256	Once in a while I feel hate toward members of my family whom I usually love.		

258	I can sleep during the day but not at night.		
259	I am sure I am been talked about.		
260	Once in a while I laugh at a dirty joke.		
262	In a group of people I would not be embarrassed to de called upon to start a discussion or give an opinion about something I know well.		
264	I have used alcohol excessively.		
265	I am likely not to speak to people until they speak to me.		
266	I have never been in trouble with the law.		
267	I have periods in which in feel usually cheerful without reason.		
269	If several people find themselves in trouble, the best thing for them to do is to agree upon a story and stick to it.		
270	It does not bother me particularly to see animals suffer.		
273	Life is strain for me much of the time.		
274	I am so touchy on some subjects that I can't talk about them.		
275	In school I found it very hard to talk in front of class.		
276	I love my mother, or (if your mother is dead) I love my mother.		
277	Even when I am with people I feel lonely much of the time.		
280	I seem to make friends about as quickly as others do.		
281	I dislike having people around me.		
282	I have been told that I walk during my sleep.		

288	My parents and my family find more faults with me than they should.		
290	I worry over money and business.		
292	The things that some of my family have done frightens me.		
295	I have never been paralyzed or had any unusual weakness of any of my muscles.		
298	Strange odours come to me at times.		
299	I cannot keep my mind on one thing.		
300	I have reason for feeling jealous of one or more members of my family.		
301	I feel anxiety about something or someone almost all the time.		
303	Most of the time I wish I were dead.		
305	I have certainly had more than my share of things to worry about.		
306	No one cares much what happens to me.		
311	I often feel as if things or not real.		
312	The only interesting part of the newspaper is the comic strips.		
316	I have strange and peculiar thoughts.		
318	I usually expect to succeed in things I do.		
319	I hear strange things when I am alone		
321	I have no dread of going into a room by myself where other people have already gathered and are talking		
323	Sometimes I enjoy hurting persons I love		

324	I can easily make other people afraid of me and sometimes do for the fun of it		
326	I have several times given up at doing a thing because I thought too little of my ability		
330	At times I am full of energy		
331	I am inclined to take things hard		
333	People say insulting and vulgar things about me		
336	Someone has control over my mind		
337	At parties I am more likely to sit by myself or just with one other person than to join in with the crowd		
338	People often disappoint me		
339	I have often felt that difficulties were piling up so high that I couldn't deal with them		
340	I love to go to dances		
341	At times my mind seems to work more slowly than usual.		
343	I enjoy children		
346	I have often met people who were supposed to be experts who were no better than I		
349	I am never happier when I am alone		
353	I enjoy social gatherings just to be with people		
355	At one or more times in my life I felt that someone was making me do things by hypnotizing me		
356	I find it hard to set aside a task that I have undertaken, even for a short time.		
359	I enjoy the excitement of a crowd		

408	I am apt to take disappointments so keenly that I cant put them out of my mind		
409	It bothers me to have someone watch me at work even though I know I can do it well.		
410	I am often so annoyed when someone tries to get ahead of me in a line of people that I speak to that person about it.		
411	At times I think I am no good at all.		
412	When I was young I often did not go to school, even though I should have gone.		
413	One or more members are very nervous.		
415	I worry quite a bit over misfortunes.		
418	It is actually all right to get around the law if you don't actually break it.		
421	I am apt to pass up something I want to de because I feel that I am not going about it in the right way.		
427	I have never seen a vision.		
428	I have several times a change of heart about my life work.		
449	Some of my family have quick tempers.		
450	I cannot do anything well.		
454	The future seems hopeless to me.		
455	The members of my family and my close relatives get along very well.		
457	People can prettily change my mind even when I have made a decision about something.		
461	It makes me angry to have people hurry me.		
462	I am not afraid of mice.		

463	Several times a week I feel as if something dreadful is about to happen.		
464	I feel tired a good deal of the time.		
466	Sometimes I am sure what other people are thinking.		
469	I sometimes feel that I am about to got o pieces.		
475	Often I get confused and forget what I wanted to say.		
476	I am very awkward and clumsy.		
478	I hate my whole family.		
479	Some people think it is hard to know me.		
480	I spend most of my spare time by myself.		
483	People do not find me attractive.		
485	I often feel that I am not as good as other people.		
486	I am very stubborn.		
490	Ghosts or spirits can influence people for good or bad.		
493	When I have a problem it helps to talk it over with someone.		
494	My main goals in life are within my reach.		
495	I believe that people should keep personal problems to themselves.		
496	I am not feeling much pressure or stress these days.		
499	I hate going to doctors even when I ma sick.		
500	Although I am not happy with my life, there is nothing I can do about it.		

501	Talking over problems and worries with someone is often more helpful than drugs or medicine.		
503	When problems need to b e solved, I usually let others take charge.		
504	I recognize several faults in myself that I will not be able to change.		
505	I am so sick of what I have to do every day that I just want to get out of all.		
506	I have recently considered killing myself.		
508	I often feel I can read other people's minds.		
512	I have a tragic loss in my life that I know I'll never get over.		
513	Sometimes I get so angry and upset that I don't know what comes over me.		
515	I am never happier than when I am by myself.		
516	My life is empty and meaningless.		
517	I find it difficult to hold own job.		
519	I get angry with myself for giving in to other people so much.		
520	Lately I have thought a lot about killing myself		
521	I like making decisions and assigning jobs to others.		
525	Everything is going on too fast around me.		
526	I know I am a burden to others.		
528	Much of the trouble I am having is due to bad luck.		
539	Lately I have lost my desire to work out my problems.		

540	I have gotten angry and broken furniture or dishes when I was drinking.		
542	I have become so angry with someone that I have felt as if I would explode.		
543	Terrible thoughts those days turn more and more to death and the life hereafter.		
548	I have been so angry sometimes that I have hurt someone in a physical fight.		
550	I have very little to do with my relatives now.		
551	I sometimes seem to hear my thoughts being spoken out loud.		
554	When my life gets difficult it just makes me want to give up.		
556	I worry a great deal about money.		
558	The only place I feel relaxed is in my own home.		
561	I usually have enough energy to do my work.		
562	It is hard for me to accept compliments.		
563	In most marriages one or both partners are unhappy.		
564	I almost never loose self-control.		
566	When I ma sad or blue, it is my work that suffers.		
567	Most married couples don't show much affection for each other.		

Section C

Please rate yourself, using the keys provided (from 0-5) since arrival from Africa to Germany: 0 = not at all; 1 = very little; 2 = sometimes; 3 = most of the time; 5 = all the time.

		0	1	2	3	4	5
1	Been Wasting away						
2	Economically improved than before						
3	Improved living standard						
4	Family Cohesion						
5	Police harassment						
6	Racial Discrimination						
7	Prejudice from Germans						
8	Prejudice from Fellow Africans						
9	Socially backward						
10	Living here is very stressful						
11	I am happy than before						
12	I am very sad						
13	I want to go back home						
14	No decent job						
15	Going through a lot of hassles						
16	I want to live here forever						
17	I am confused						
18	Regretted coming here						
19	Equal opportunities to job and health care						
20	Confronted with so many problems						

Section D

Here we briefly describe the "German person" or the "German people". Please read each description and think about how much the German is or not like you. Put an X in the box to the right or Circle the number that shows how much the person in the description is like you.

Please use the following key: 6 = very much like me; 5 = like me; 4 = somewhat like me; 3 = a little like me; 2 = not like me; 1 = not like me at all.

HOW MUCH LIKE YOU IS THIS PERSON?

1.	Thinking up new ideas and being creative is important to him/her. He/she likes to do things in her own original way. (SD)	1	2	3	4	5	6
2.	It is important to him/her to be rich. He/she wants to have a lot of money and expensive things. (PO)	1	2	3	4	5	6
3.	He/she thinks it is important that every person in the world be treated equally. He/she believes everyone should have equal opportunities in life. (UN)	1	2	3	4	5	6
4.	It's important to him/her to show his/her abilities. He/she wants people to admire what he/she does. (AC)	1	2	3	4	5	6
5.	It is important to him/her to live in secure surroundings. He/she avoids anything that might endanger his/her safety. (SE)	1	2	3	4	5	6
6.	He/she likes surprises and is always looking for new things to do. He/she thinks it is important to do lots of different things in life. (ST)	1	2	3	4	5	6

7.	He/she believes that people should do what they're told. He/she thinks people should follow rules at all times, even when no-one is watching. (CO)	1	2	3	4	5	6
8.	It is important to him/her to listen to people who are different from him/her. Even when he/she disagrees with them, he/she still wants to understand them. (UN)	1	2	3	4	5	6
9.	It is important to him/her to be humble and modest. He/she tries not to draw attention to herself. (TR)	1	2	3	4	5	6
10.	Having a good time is important to him/her. He/she likes to "spoil" him/herself. (HE)	1	2	3	4	5	6
11.	It is important to him/her to make his/her own decisions about what he/she does. He/she likes to be free and not depend on others. (SD)	1	2	3	4	5	6
12.	It's very important to him/her to help the people around him/her. He/she wants to care for their wellbeing. (BE)	1	2	3	4	5	6
13.	Being very successful is important to him/her. He/she hopes people will recognize his/her achievements. (AC)	1	2	3	4	5	6
14.	It is important to him/her that the government insure his/her safety against all threats. He/she wants the state to be strong so it can defend its citizens. (SE)	1	2	3	4	5	6
15.	He/she looks for adventures and likes to take risks. He/she wants to have an exciting life. (ST)	1	2	3	4	5	6

16.	It is important to him/her always to behave properly. He/she wants to avoid doing anything people would say is wrong. (CO)	1	2	3	4	5	6
17.	It is important to him/her to get respect from others. He/she wants people to do what he/she says. (PO)	1	2	3	4	5	6
18.	It is important to him/her to be loyal to his/her friends. He/she wants to devote him/herself to people close to him/her. (BE)	1	2	3	4	5	6
19.	He/she strongly believes that people should care for nature. Looking after the environment is important to him/her. (UN)	1	2	3	4	5	6
20.	Tradition is important to him/her. He/she tries to follow the customs handed down by his/her religion or his/her family. (TR)	1	2	3	4	5	6
21.	He/she seeks every chance he/she can to have fun. It is important to him/her to do things that give him/her pleasure. (HE)	1	2	3	4	5	6

Thank you for your cooperation!

Epilogue

Idemudia and Boehnke have provided us with empirical evidence on the mental health, acculturative stress, and value preferences in a small but very special sample of African immigrants to Germany. Their research is unique in two ways: they report on a study of immigrants that was carried out in a receiving society that is not all that common as a destination for African migrants; and their sample also includes illegal immigrants and imprisoned migrants. This study was only possible because the first author is an African who was able to access fellow Africans in difficult life situations. However, some potential study participants seemingly did refuse to fill in the questionnaire, because they thought of the first author as a secret agent either of the German or of African governments.

The instrument used to survey African immigrants in Germany had three components. It included a lengthy selection of items from one of the most widely used clinical psychological instruments on mental health deficiencies, the Minnesota Multiphasic Personality Inventory (MMPI). The instrument dates back to the late 1930s, but they used in its revised version (MMPI-2; introduced some 20 years ago). The study also included an ad hoc measure of acculturative stress, and a variant of Schwartz's 21-item Portrait Value Questionnaire (PVQ). The latter instrument was modeled after the version used in the European Social Survey. It used an instruction that forced participants to report their own value preferences in contrast to what they were instructed to see as 'the typical German:' The protagonist of the portraits presented in the PVQ was designated as a German.

Results of the study certainly do not provide grounds for optimism. The findings are difficult to assess from a clinical psychological point of view because there is no standardization available for MMPI-2 scores for Africa in general, or for African migrants in an aversive receiving society such as Germany in particular. The study makes it clear that the African immigrant population in Germany is not all that well-off with respect to their mental health. Even though the study can certainly not be interpreted in any epidemiological manner, being a snowball sample of small size, it seems obvious that the respondents have high scores on at least three of the MMPI clinical subscales: depression, somatic and psychosomatic medical problems, and psychological dysfunction in work performance.

The acculturative stress measure that the authors used can obviously be criticized for its ad hoc character. At the same time it must be applauded for its ecological validity: All items originate from focus group discussions with African immigrants in Germany. The language used in the items in their original form closely resembled the Creole English that was prevalent in the focus group discussions, and that is widely spoken in Anglophone Africa. What becomes evident is that African immigrants report high levels of stress originating from two possible sources (Berry, 2006)[14]. First, they are overwhelmed with daily hassles. For those with non-legalized status, this adds to the experience of stress, because beyond struggling with everyday life in an aversive environment they have to uphold their 'secrecy.' Second, the high levels of stress may also have predominantly cultural roots, in that people who have grown up in cultures that typically differ from Germany in perceptions of time, efficiency, and *Ordnung* may experience the typical German lifestyle as stressful in and of itself. Part of both sources of stress is, the experience of racism in Germany; this was obviously a major stressor that came out quite clearly, both in the Migrant Attitude Scale as well as in initial open questions.

Value preferences of African migrants in Germany are difficult to assess given that no comparison data exist and that a peculiar format of assessment was used, which asked participants to report their own value preferences in contrast to the average German. However, with some reservation it can be said that Africans in Germany have higher preferences than Germans for security values (ranking #1 among the surveyed Africans, but typically ranking #5 or 6 in German samples) and for power values (ranking #6 among Africans, but typically ranking #9 or 10 in German samples). These discrepant value preferences are likely to add another component to Africans perceiving themselves as 'Aliens in *Deutschland*', and to serve as a cultural source of stress.

Yet more interesting than the descriptive findings commented upon above are the multivariate results Idemudia and Boehnke present. Their most worrisome result is that acculturative stress increases with the duration of stay. Much research suggests that in general acculturative stress should vary over time, with an increase in the early years, followed by a decline (Sam & Berry, 2006). This is not the case among African immigrants to Germany. They suffer from higher levels of stress the longer they have stayed in Germany, even when the result is partialled for possible age effect. Idemudia

[14] References for the epilogue are incorporated in the general reference list of the volume.

and Boehnke see the trap of a double bind here in that a higher percentage of the study participants report that their economic situation has clearly improved compared to the situation they were in before migration, while at the same time they report increased stress levels with longer stays in Germany. This paradox forces the migrants to stay in an environment that they experience as highly stressful if they do not want to risk undermining their economic existence.

No wonder that in this situation the relationship between levels of self-reported acculturative stress and overall mental health is high, higher than in most other studies. Both acculturative stress levels and the level of perceived German racism are closely and independently related to overall mental health. The strength of the relationship between acculturative stress and the overall poor mental health score may be inflated somewhat by conceptual overlaps in the measures of both, but they are certainly quite high. What is yet more important is that duration of stay in Germany, gender, family fragmentation and economic need as a migration motivation have no direct relationship with mental health. The sometimes strong impact of these factors on mental health is fully mediated by acculturative stress: Those migrants, who have stayed in Germany longer, who are women, are separated from their spouses, and came for economic reasons experience a higher level of acculturative stress, which in turn predicts a substantial proportion of variance in poor mental health. Economic refugees furthermore report substantially higher levels of perceived German racism, another noteworthy predictor of poor mental health. Only chronological age (the older the better one's mental health) and having had some secondary schooling (but not more), stand in a direct relationship with mental health. Such a finding might suggest that there could be selection effects in play, namely that a major proportion of those coming with a lower level of education may have had mental health problems already at home. Nevertheless, the results of Idemudia and Boehnke's study suggest that a longer stay in Germany, family fragmentation, and coming primarily for economic reasons serve as independent risk factors for acculturative stress and (in part) perceived racism, and consequentially poor mental health among Africans in Germany.

What serves as a protective factor? It is not so much relative economic success in Germany (as reported by the study participants), but is most likely 'eaten up' in its possible positive effect by the precariousness of the job situation in Germany. As often found in research (e.g., Aycan & Berry, 1996), African immigrants to Germany tend to be economically successful in comparison to the time before migration, but the jobs they hold are clearly experienced as indecent; this probably is causing some of the work interference-type psychological dysfunctions detected by the pertinent MMPI scale. The only protection factor against acculturative stress reported in the study is holding value preferences similar to those common in German culture. In an interesting post hoc interpretation Idemudia and Boehnke see 'Germanized' values as a proxy for what I have in my work (Berry, 2005) described as the acculturation style of *integration*. They argue that Blacks in Germany have no chance to validly choose *assimilation* as their preferred acculturation style, because of their skin color. They also are highly unlikely to take the *marginalization* trajectory, because the African community is very tightly knit in a Diaspora setting like Germany. This means that they tend to have only two options, *separation* and integration. One operationalization of the acculturation style of separation would then be holding tight to African value preferences (e.g., high power values), whereas taking up German mainstream values would serve as an operationalization of preference for an acculturation style of integration. This finding is, of course, not tested by Idemudia and Boehnke's study. It would need further research urgently, but is an indication for the validity of the hypothesis that a value-related person-environment fit fosters well-being.

All in all, the authors make a strong case for the difficult situation of Blacks in the Diaspora, by documenting the serious mental-health problems that became obvious in the survey undertaken.

Dealing with these results is, of course, not so much a psychological question as a political one. Yes, offering increased family counseling to African migrants in Germany is an important potential remedy against family fragmentation, but it does not serve as a strong protection against the deteriorating mental health of long-time African residents of Germany. What can only help there is an increase in basic hospitality: Making African immigrants welcome in their new home is what is needed, not a tendency towards a bulwark Europe, nor an ethnically clean, homogeneous Germany. This openness to the 'other', and a willingness to change, are essential components of the European Union Basic Common Principles for integration in Europe: "Integration is a dynamic, two-way process of mutual accommodation by all immigrants and residents of Member States" (EU, 2005). In my view, following this principle would be beneficial not only for Africans in Germany, but to the whole of German society.

At the same time there is a need for an investment by the Western world in ‘decent’ jobs in Africa. The critical discrepancy between Africans not being able to find decent jobs in Germany, but at the same time still being better off than before migration, needs to be narrowed in a concerted action by countries of the West along with the nations of Africa.

John W. Berry
Queen’s University
Kingston, ON, Canada
September 2009

The Authors

Erhabor Sunday Idemudia is a Clinical Psychologist, who has a double appointment as Full Professor in South Africa, both at North-West University at Mafikeng and at the University of Limpopo, Turfloop Campus, where he had also been Associate Professor since 2006. He earned his PhD in Clinical Psychology in 1995 from the University of Ibadan, Nigeria. Earlier he has held positions as Lecturer and Senior Lecturer at the University of Ibadan and the University of Namibia in Windhoek, and as Associate Professor at the University of Ibadan. He has been awarded fellowships from the University of California, Los Angeles (UCLA), from Alexander von Humboldt Foundation (AvH), Germany; from the Conseil pour le Développement de la Recherche en Sciences Sociales, Dakar, Senegal (fellow and laureate), from San José State University (Salzburg Fellow), from the Centre for African Studies, London (Leventis Fellow), and from the Albert Ellis Institute. He is Secretary-General of African Chapter of the World Council for Psychotherapy. Professor Idemudia also serves as Associate Editor of the Journal of Child and Adolescent Mental Health, the International Journal of Human Ecology, and the Journal of Studies on Ethno-Medicine, and is Board Member and former Vice Director and Senior Consultant Clinical Psychologist of the Catholic Consulting and Therapeutic Centre, Benin City, Nigeria. He has published widely in books and peer-reviewed academic journals. Teaching and research interests include migration and cross-cultural issues in psychology, the psychology of distressed and vulnerable groups, sexuality including HIV/AIDS, and trauma studies.

Klaus Boehnke is a Professor of Social Science Methodology at Jacobs University Bremen, Germany, since 2002, and Vice Dean of the Bremen International Graduate School of Social Sciences (BIGSSS). He earned his PhD in Psychology in 1985 from Berlin University of Technology. Earlier he has held positions as Lecturer and Research Associate at Berlin University of Technology, Assistant and Associate Professor at the Free University of Berlin, and Full Professor at the Department of Sociology of Chemnitz University of Technology, Germany. He has also held visiting appointments at the Australian National University in Canberra (1987), the University of Toronto (1997/8), and the National University of Singapore (2008/9). Professor Boehnke has served the International Association for Cross-Cultural Psychology (IACCP) as its Secretary-General from 2000-2008, and is President of the Division of Political Psychology of the International Association of Applied Psychology (IAAP). He has acted as reviewer for some ten national and international science funding organizations and over 40 academic journals, and has published and edited 20 books and special issues of peer-reviewed journals, and over 250 pieces of academic writing in peer-reviewed journals and as book chapters. He mostly teaches statistical methodology to diverse social science student audiences. His research interests lie in the field of political socialization, including studies on values and values transmission in the family and under conditions of social change.

John Winthrop Berry, the author of this volume's epilogue, is Professor Emeritus at Queen's University in Kingston, ON, Canada, where he has held consecutive professorial positions since 1969. He has received his PhD from the University of Edinburgh in 1966 and has held his first academic position at the University of Sydney immediately thereafter. Professor Berry is acclaimed as the nestor of modern acculturation research and has published widely in the field. He has also been Secretary-General and President of the International Association for Cross-Cultural Psychology (IACCP) and is that organization's Honorary Fellow. As a Professor Emeritus he continues to engage extensively in comparative acculturation research and has recently been co-editor (with David Sam) of the Cambridge Handbook of Acculturation Psychology.

www.ingramcontent.com/pod-product-compliance
Ingram Content Group UK Ltd.
Pitfield, Milton Keynes, MK11 3LW, UK
UKHW021842100926
8556IPUK00019B/991

9 783631 599754